Hashimotos

Cure Hashimoto's Thyroiditis Once and for All!

New Hashimoto's Diet for a Healthy Life

Veronica Baruwal

Veronica Baruwal

© **Copyright 2015 - All rights reserved.**

In no way is it legal to reproduce, duplicate, or transmit any part of this document in either electronic means or in printed format. Recording of this publication is strictly prohibited and any storage of this document is forbidden unless with written permission from the publisher. All rights reserved.

The information provided herein is stated to be truthful and consistent, in that any liability, in terms of inattention or otherwise, by any usage or abuse of any policies, processes, or directions contained within is the solitary and utter responsibility of the recipient reader. Under no circumstances will any legal responsibility or blame be held against the publisher for any reparation, damages, or monetary loss due to the information herein, either directly or indirectly.

Respective authors own all copyrights not held by the publisher.

Legal Notice:

Veronica Baruwal

This book is copyright protected. This is only for personal use. You cannot amend, distribute, sell, use, quote or paraphrase any part or the content within this book without the consent of the author or copyright owner. Legal action will be pursued if this is breached.

Disclaimer Notice:

Please note the information contained within this document is for educational and entertainment purposes only. Every attempt has been made to provide accurate, up to date and reliable complete information. No warranties of any kind are expressed or implied. Readers acknowledge that the author is not engaging in the rendering of legal, financial, medical or professional advice.

Table of Contents

Introduction 9

Chapter 1: Thyroid Gland 11

Chapter 2: Hashimoto's Thyroiditis 15

Chapter 3: Causes of Hashimoto's Thyroiditis 27

Chapter 4: Diagnosis of Hashimoto's Disease 35

Chapter 5: How to Prevent Hashimoto's Thyroiditis? 43

Chapter 6: Hashimoto's Disease and Pregnancy 53

Chapter 7: Treatments for Hashimoto's 61

Chapter 8: Hashimoto's Disease and Diet 69

Chapter 9: Paleolithic Diet and Recipes 77
    La Piperade 83
    Crepes 85
    Apricot Pesto Chicken with Basil 87
    Potato Salad Packing with Probiotics 89
    Avocado Cucumber Summer Cold Soup 91
    Almond Bread 93

Dill, Asparagus, and Fennel Soup 95
Apple and Zucchini Pancakes Made with Almond Flour 98
Quinoa with Nuts and Goji Berries 100
Celery root and Squash Soup 102
Raw Marinated Mushrooms 105
Warm Oysters with Vinaigrette 106
Grill Zucchini Hummus 108
Apricot Power Bars 110
Egg Muffins Delight 112
Delicious Breakfast Hash 114
Fruit and chicken salad 116
Delicious Pepper Chicken Stir-fry 118
Tuna Avocado Wraps in Lettuce 119
Baked Salmon in Maple Syrup 121
Southwest Omelets 123
Sweet Potato Hash 125
Chocolate Doughnuts with Coffee 127
Turkey Salad with Avocado and Lettuce 129
Easy Pan Chicken With Green Peas and Butternut Squash 131
Zesty Salmon with Parsley and Dill 133
Delicious Cornbread Muffins 135
Fried Okra in Pork Batter 137

Grilled Steak 139
Sausage and Asparagus Casserole 141
Delicious Tomato and Dill Frittata 143
Prosciutto Peach Salad with an Arugula Dressing 145
Chicken Enchilada Bake 147
Sausage Frittata 149
Delicious Italian Meatballs 151
Zucchini Patties 153

Chapter 10: Hashimoto's Disease and Workout 155
    Hashimoto's thyroiditis and yoga 157

Chapter 11: Dealing with Hashimoto's Thyroiditis as a Vegan 160

Chapter 12: Home Remedies for Hashimoto's Thyroiditis 167

Chapter 13: Myths Associated with Hashimoto's Thyroiditis 177

Chapter 14: Tips and Points to be Noted 185

Conclusion 199

Veronica Baruwal

Introduction

Our world today is fast paced. It is full of competition and a thirst to gain more and more from life. Unfortunately, due to this type of lifestyle, we tend to neglect our health, despite it being much more important than any kind of wealth or monetary gains. Due to this constant neglect of health, a lot of new diseases and disorders keep cropping up. These diseases can not only ruin your physical health, they can wreck your mental health as well. One such disorder is the Hashimoto's Thyroiditis.

Over the past few years Hashimoto's thyroiditis has been diagnosed more often and thus has taken a center stage. Hashimoto's thyroiditis is an autoimmune disease where the immune cells of the body start to attack the body's own cells.

Veronica Baruwal

The thyroid gland is the organ affected and it suffers extremely thus making this disorder quite a painful ordeal

In this book, I will talk about the structure and functions of the thyroid gland in order to better understand why this disease is so dangerous. I will also provide you with the detailed study about what Hashimoto's thyroiditis is all about. It will include the symptoms, diagnosis, and treatment of this disease, along with a diet plan that will aid in controlling and curing this disease. Thus this book will prove to be a definitive guide for you on Hashimoto's thyroiditis.

Thank you for choosing this book, **Hashimoto's: Ultimate Guide to Cure Hashimoto's Thyroiditis, Hashimoto's Diet.** I hope that you benefit from the book and that it helps you manage this disorder.

Good luck.

Chapter 1
Thyroid Gland

Before discussing any disorder or disease that affects a certain body part or organ, it is vital to understand the workings of the particular organ it affects and to know some basic facts about it. In this case, it is quite necessary to know what the thyroid gland is, where it is situated and what it does.

The thyroid gland is not only the largest endocrinal glands of the body, but it is also one of the most important ones. The thyroid gland is in the neck, in front of the trachea and just behind the esophagus. There are two lobes in the thyroid gland; the right lobe and the left lobe. Both of these are connected together by an isthmus. The lobes of the thyroid glands are pear shaped. The thyroid gland normally weighs 12 to 20 grammes, contains a high amount of vessels, and has a soft consistency. There are four parathyroid glands, which are located behind the thyroid gland, and they produce the parathyroid hormone which helps in secreting and regulating the levels of calcium in an individual's body.

Functions of the thyroid gland

We just learned about the structure of the thyroid gland so now it is essential to understand what exactly the function of the thyroid gland is and why it is supposedly one of the most important organs of the human body.

The thyroid gland is very important because it is primarily responsible for the production of two important hormones, thyroxin (T4) and Triiodothyronine (T3). These hormones act through the nuclear receptors and play a very important role for cell differentiation during growth and help to maintain thermogenic and metabolic homeostasis in the adult. The disorders that affect the thyroid gland are usually the result of an autoimmune process where either there is a simulative increase in producing thyroid hormones or there is a systematic glandular destruction that results in the deficiency of the hormone. Both of these conditions are quite harmful.

Veronica Baruwal

Chapter 2
Hashimoto's Thyroiditis

As was said previously, the thyroid gland is affected mostly by autoimmune disorders that can cause a lot of harm to the body. One such disorder that is infamous nowadays due to its spread is the Hashimoto's Thyroiditis. In this chapter, I will cover some of the major introductory facts regarding Hashimoto's Thyroiditis.

As was previously explained, Hashimoto's Thyroiditis is an autoimmune disorder where the body's own immune cells destroy the tissues. It is also commonly known as chronic lymphocytic thyroiditis. Thyroiditis means inflammation of the thyroid gland. Hypothyroidism is one of the main results of Hashimoto's Thyroiditis.

Prevalence

Hashimoto's Thyroiditis is gaining recognition in the medical field due to its increased prevalence. Many people now are suffering from a disorder which was relatively unknown some years ago. Hashimoto's thyroiditis has a higher rate of occurrence in males than females. Research has shown that the mean annual incidence rate of this disorder is up to 4 per 1000 women and 1 per 1000 males. This disease is more commonly seen in Japanese individuals. This is thought to be due to genetic and hereditary factors and also due to increased exposure to iodine diet.

The average age of this disease is about 60 years and the risk of contracting this disease increases as the individual is getting older; thus the elderly are highly susceptible to this disorder.

Clinical manifestation

One important factor you must know is that it is a slow disorder. The symptoms of this disease are slow and gradual, but very adverse. Individuals can develop symptoms that are mild to major in a very short period of time. The individual suffering from Hashimoto's Thyroiditis may go to the physician with just goiter rather than any symptoms of hypothyroidism. You may already have the disorder and not even notice any symptoms. There are individuals who do not experience any symptoms even when they are diagnosed with Hashimoto's disease. The goiter may be large in size, irregular in shape and firm in its consistency. Initially the goiter may be painless, but over the years, if it is left untreated, it can lead to an increased pressure on the esophagus, which makes it difficult for the individual to swallow food and thus making it a very painful and uncomfortable ordeal.

There are individuals who develop no symptoms or only minor symptoms; this is called sub clinical hypothyroidism or mild hypothyroidism. Those who develop a wide range of full-grown symptoms are said to be suffering from clinical hypothyroidism. Thus there are various different symptoms and forms of this disorder.

This disease manifests its symptoms on varied organs and parts of the body and usually doesn't concentrate on one part. It targets anything and everything. The thyroid gland is not the only organ which deteriorates as a result; many of the organs of the body can suffer the effects of this disease as well. Many of these organs are highly important to maintain the general wear and tear of the body. Here I have listed many of the symptoms that you may experience with this disorder. The symptoms are divided according to the place or organ they can affect.

On the skin

This condition can easily affect the skin. It can become dry and patched. The skin tightens which leads to increased difficulty with moving muscles. There can be a noticeable decrease in perspiration and the epidermis layer of the skin can thin.

On the nails

The nails are affected by this disorder as well. In fact, you could even diagnose yourself if you observe your nails daily and note any sudden change in them. This sudden change can be in their texture, color, shine etc. Their hardness is also an important factor. People who suffer from

Hashimoto's Thyroiditis often notice that the nails become weak and brittle and break easily, and that they lose their shine and look dull.

On the hair

Hair is also targeted by Hashimoto's disorder. Like nails, you can observe your hair to keep an eye on your health. If you notice any sudden change in the quality, texture, color, strength etc. of your hair you should consult your doctor. In case of Hashimoto's, the hair becomes dry and brittle, making it very difficult for an individual to manage it. Hair may fall out easily, resulting in bald patches in mild cases but also alopecia when the case worsens. Also some individuals note that their hair turns grey sooner due to this disorder.

On the face

The face can become bloated with swollen eyelids. You may also notice non-pitting edema, which is the bloating of the body due to accumulation of liquids that indent on pressure, on the hands and legs of the individual suffering from this disease.

Sleep disorders

The person may also have sleep related issues, such as insomnia and disturbed sleep. Due to inadequate sleep, individuals may have mood swings. Inadequate sleep is also harmful as it can affect your every day life. It can ruin your daily schedule, harm your concentration power and disrupt your body functions. Lack of sleep is harmful for your overall health. You may become fatigued, irritable, etc. because of irregular sleep patterns.

Hormonal and reproductive issues

The functioning of the thyroid gland is essential for the production and regulation of female hormones, which are necessary for menstruation and ovulation. If these hormones are not regulated properly it can cause lot problems for those who menstruate. People suffering from Hashimoto's disease often suffer from menstrual disorders like oligomenorrhea, which refers to scanty or infrequent menses. Also, in a chronic, long-standing disease condition, there may be amenorrhea, where there is complete absence of periods. Some individuals also complain of menorrhagia, where there is heavy bleeding during periods. there can also be an increase in premenstrual symptoms such as extreme pain in the lower abdomen before menses, severe mood swings, tenderness of the breasts, increased food cravings, etc. All of these cause major discomfort and can negatively impact those who suffer with Hashimoto's.

Those who suffer with the disease may also find it difficult to become pregnant even when at the peak of their ovulation cycle as the disease can affect fertility. In the rare situation of a sufferer successfully conceiving, the pregnancy will usually result in a miscarriage.

Sexual deficiency

This disorder can also affect the sexual prowess of the patient. Many sufferers have reported a loss of libido due to the disorder. This reduce in sex drive and thus makes sex boring or undesirable.

Gastrointestinal complaints

A negative effect can be seen on the digestive as well as excretory system as a result of this disorder. This disorder affects the metabolism of the patient which thus affects the digestion and also the excretory system. Constipation and IBS are also common in patients.

On the muscles

As said earlier, this disorder can affect the tissues present in human body. Thus people who suffer from this disease get tired very easily because the capacity of their muscles decreases. Even if the person does little work, he or she may get tired and fatigued. This tiredness is also associated with muscle pain, soreness and cramps that are severe in nature.

The disorder also affects the circulatory system as well as the blood present in the body. It can cause various malfunctions such as anemia.

Cold intolerance

People who suffer from this disease report not being able to bear the cold. Even a little drop in the temperature can affect them negatively. This is because their hands and feet cannot retain heat well, giving them the sensation of always being cold. Thus you may find them wearing warm clothes and gloves even at the most inappropriate occasions.

On the brain

The brain is certainly the most important organ of the body. This too can be severely affected because of the disorder in various ways. There can be a noticeable decrease in the concentration prowess of the person suffering as they may find it difficult to focus on a particular subject for a long period of time. This reduces the subject's productivity as they cannot concentrate and focus on their tasks.

Along with concentration, the disorder can also cause many memory related problems. Initially there is weakness of memory and forgetfulness, and if this is left untreated it can result in long-term memory loss. This also reduces the work efficiency of the patients.

The disorder also slows the person's brain functions and other activities. The patients often think very sluggishly, often taking a lot of time to think and react. Severe depression has also been noticed in long, untreated cases. Lower IQ levels are found in children who are born with hypothyroid. Thus this disorder not only interferes in the physical aspects of the brain but also the psychological aspects as well.

Obesity

Sufferers often complain about either gaining too much weight, or complain about the difficulty in shedding those extra pounds. Despite the fact that poor appetite tends to be a symptom of Hashimoto's, sufferers gain weight easily. The metabolism of these patients is sluggish, which in turn results in weight gain. Because sufferers also lack energy, they can hardly exercise and so find it difficult to lose weight by exercising.

On the heart

As said earlier, the circulatory system is affected by this disorder. There is a notable decrease in the myocardial contractility and this in turn decreases the pulse rate count. Patients also frequently complain of some pain in the chest.

On the speech

As the brain is affected, various sensory organs or senses are affected too. The voice is one such sense. The voice slowly gets hoarse and speech becomes slow and clumsy. This is a major tell-tale sign that there is something wrong that needs your immediate attention

On children

Although autoimmune diseases are not very common in children, Hashimoto's can affect children. If a child contracts an autoimmune disease, there is a considerable delay in the growth of the child. The growth cycle of the overall body is affected quite brutally. The facial maturation is very slow and there is a delay in teething too. The muscular reflexes of the child become slow and muscle swelling occurs. If the disease occurs before 3 years of age, the child may also suffer from impaired intellectual development.

Low immunity level

The immunity levels of these individuals is very low, because their own body cells, which are supposed to provide them immunity from a variety of diseases, are busy attacking the healthy tissue. They suffer from a large amount of infectious diseases, especially from respiratory diseases like the cold flu, and cold and cough. The recovery from such diseases is very slow and with each bout of the disease there is an increase in the severity of the disease. It is highly important for these patients to protect themselves from any kind of illness as even the common cold can wreck havoc on their body.

Until now we have seen the various symptoms that can affect the various organs of the patient. As you can see, this disorder can cause a variety of problems for sufferers.

Chapter 3
Causes of Hashimoto's Thyroiditis

Although our world is modern and technologically advanced, there are still many mysteries around us that have yet to be solved. Most of these mysteries concern medical science and they have baffled doctors and scientists from a long time. Hashimoto's is one of those medical mysteries.

Even with so much medical knowledge and rapidly developing technology, no one knows the exact cause of Hashimoto's Thyroiditis. There is no exact reason or cause available as to why this disorder occurs. But, after thorough research, doctors have penned down a list of known factors, which are considered to be the main causes for the development of Hashimoto's disease in individuals. Genetic and environmental conditions are the two important factors that work together.

The body has a system which has a responsibility to protect and save the body from harmful foreign viruses and bacteria. This system is known as the immune system. This system is one of the rare boons that Mother Nature has bestowed upon us. But, in this disease, for reasons unknown, the immune system fights the body's own cells and destroys its healthy tissues and thus becomes a curse. Instead of destroying the unwanted foreign bacteria that has invaded the body, the disease goes on to destroy the body itself.

Let us have a look at some of the alleged reasons why this disorder occurs.

Family history

Individuals who have members of their family suffering from Hashimoto's disease or any other type of autoimmune disorder are more prone to developing this disease. It is not exactly hereditary but those who have had family members with this disorder should beware of it.

Individuals who already suffer from an auto immune disease

It is a common occurrence that if a person is suffering from one disease or disorder belonging to a certain organ, they may suffer or contract another disorder or disease of the same organ. Similar is the case of Hashimoto's disease. This disease is commonly seen in individuals who are already suffering from a pre existing autoimmune condition. This disorder attacks the immune system, it weakens it considerably and thus the patient is at a high risk. Their immune system is not functioning properly, so they are more likely to develop another autoimmune disease condition. They could also previously suffer from diseases like rheumatoid arthritis and type 1 diabetes, which are some of the most commonly observed autoimmune disease conditions in people around the world. Patients suffering from these diseases are quite susceptible to Hashimoto's.

People who suffer from these autoimmune diseases should undergo regular check-ups for Hashimoto's Thyroiditis, since they are the ones who are at most risk of suffering from Hashimoto's disease. Early diagnosis will help you in early detection and so one can start with immediate management and treatment without much delay. Remember, prevention is always better than a cure; a stitch in time can save nine.

Genetic cause

It is strongly believed that there is a genetic link for Hashimoto's disease. This has been scientifically studied and results have found that a specific gene, HLA-DR5, is noticed to be present in all the people who suffer from Hashimoto's disease. This genetic trait is more commonly seen in monozygotic twins. It is possible that this disorder may be a genetic disorder.

Environmental factors

Our environment is made of living and non-living things that surround us. It has a great influence on us. Unfortunately, due to many modern and technological developments, the environment has been suffering. This is because of the self-centered humanism which has seen a wide spread neglect towards the environment, other people, other species during recent times and is destroying the environment. Unfortunately for us, these dangerous alterations of the environmental system are extremely harmful and as human beings are a part of the environment, this affects us as well.

There are many harmful effects of environmental imbalance. It can even cause a lot of diseases and disorders. Hashimoto's disorder is thought to possibly be a result of environmental imbalances.

Environmental triggers play a very important role in the development of Hashimoto's disease. These factors are living factors as well as non-living factors. Out of the living factors, bacterial and viral infections are the most commonly known cause for the disease.

There are many non-living factors as well. The air is polluted with a lot of toxins, pesticides and other chemicals because of the ever-rising number of industries and the use of chemicals in almost everything, from cooking to agriculture. Many times the chemicals used in these processes form a residue which then gets spread through the environment, especially in the air, thus polluting it. We are all breathing this polluted air every day and we all are at risk of contracting this disease. Certain areas, such as urban areas, are more polluted than the rural areas and thus the level of toxins is higher in the cities compared to the countryside. These toxins and chemicals that we breathe enter into our body, enter the system and unbalance the hormonal activity that is already taking place in our body. This causes a major shift that is responsible for developing autoimmune diseases, such as Hashimoto's Thyroiditis. These chemicals and toxins can also interfere with your other vital systems and can be temporary or even permanent.

Mercury and fluoride also work as endocrinal enemies. If you have more than the required quantities of mercury and fluoride in your body, it hampers the normal endocrinal activity. Fluoride is mostly present in water and toothpaste that we use on a daily basis, so it is very important to check the contents of the toothpaste before we purchase to avoid unnecessary problems. It is also necessary to get your water checked regularly for impurities.

Stress

Another harmful result of the technological and industrial boom is the rising levels of tension and stress. Due to the unbelievable level of competition and struggle that is steadfastly becoming the norm of the day, stress levels have been rising like the rate of inflation. People as young as 5 years of age suffer from stress. This results in a variety of health problems, including Hashimoto's. Too much mental stress is not very good for your health. This stress can be one of the reasons why there is an insufficient conversion of T4 to T3, thus making you susceptible to this disease. Stress also leads to other disorders and diseases and thus it is advised that one should try to stay away from stress as much as possible.

Pregnancy

The body goes through many changes during pregnancy, both mental and physical. There are a lot of hormonal fluctuations taking place within the body but unfortunately these fluctuations can cause problems. At times, immunity can also decrease, making the body more susceptible to illness. The risk of developing this disease is also high after pregnancy when the body is weak both from supporting the fetus and from labor.

Deficiency

Deficiency is the lack of certain elements. In terms of the body, deficiency refers to a lack of certain nutritional elements. As a sudden increase in the levels of some elements is harmful for the body, in the same manner, a sudden decrease in the levels of certain elements can be harmful too. In this case low Iodine intake in meals and selenium deficiency play a major role in developing this condition.

Chapter 4
Diagnosis of Hashimoto's Disease

Diagnosing a disease or disorder is definitely taking the first step towards treating it. Diagnosing a disorder can be difficult because, even in this modern and technologically advanced era, the issue of wrong diagnosis remains. This wrong diagnosis can prove to be a very harmful thing and can even prove to be fatal. Thus it is very important to diagnose this condition correctly.

There are many ways of diagnosing Hashimoto's Thyroiditis. It may be detected by undergoing a physical examination or by noticing the various signs and symptoms. But if you want a thorough confirmation that you have this particular disease, the best way is to get yourself clinically diagnosed by a physician. This is the best way to confirm the status of your health. It is always better that you visit your family doctor, and they will help you further by asking you to do certain laboratory investigations. This may be expensive, but it's better to be safe than sorry. Remember, prevention is always better than a cure. There are many tests prescribed for the diagnosis of Hashimoto's disorder.

The tests include:

- Thyroid stimulating test (TSH)
- Anti thyroid antibodies test
- Free T4 test

Now let us have a closer look at each of these tests to understand what exactly is diagnosed in these tests. First let's check out what is TSH.

Thyroid stimulating hormone

TSH is one of the most common tests prescribed for the diagnosis of Hashimoto's disorder. TSH is Thyroid Stimulating Hormone test. TSH is a very common blood test and is the most essential test asked to be conducted on patients who have thyroid related complaints. Thyroid stimulating hormone or Thyrotrophic is a hormone, which is synthesized and secreted by the anterior pituitary, which helps in regulating the endocrinal functions of the thyroid gland. TSH levels are commonly tested in patients suspected of having hypothyroidism.

The decrease in thyroid gland secretion is immediately detected by the pituitary gland and, in order to correct this situation, the pituitary gland secretes a large amount of the thyroid-stimulating hormone, to help stimulate the thyroid gland to produce more hormones.

The main aim of performing thyroid stimulating test is to know whether the TSH levels are within normal limits or not. The standard normal range varies from 0.35-5.5 milli units per liter, but at times the range varies in some individuals.

So in simple words if your TSH level is higher than normal, it means that your brain is getting a signal that your thyroid gland is producing inadequate amounts of hormones for normal functions to take place in the body and so, in response, it needs a bit of stimulation. So, you can detect the abnormalities present in the thyroid gland quite easily with this test.

Anti thyroid antibodies test

The second important and commonly prescribed test is the anti thyroid antibody test. Anti thyroid antibody test or anti thyroglobulin test is a very useful test for confirmation and detection of Hashimoto's thyroiditis.

As I have already mentioned, Hashimoto's thyroiditis is an autoimmune disorder, wherein the immune system does not function in harmony with the body. The immune system, which is the most responsible component of the body and helps to protect and destroy the various unwanted and harmful substances in the body, abandons its job and does not attack these harmful substances; rather it attacks and destroys the other healthy tissues of the body and thus becomes a saboteur.

When the cells from the immune system attack the healthy thyroid gland tissue, it produces antibodies. Thus, these anti thyroids antibodies tests help in detecting these antibodies in the thyroid gland, and measure the anti body levels. So, the test is most important for the detection of this disease. The normal range varies from 1-20 micro grams per liter. If the antibodies, or rather the rate of antibodies, is less than the said number then it can be clearly seen that something is wrong.

Free T4

This is another test that can be used to determine whether a person has the Hashimoto's disease or not. T4, thyroxin or tetraiodothyronine is the most essential test your doctor will suggest you to investigate in order to diagnose Hashimoto's disease. T4 is a type of thyroid hormone and it is one of the most important hormones secreted by the follicular cells of the thyroid gland. Free T4 is a more valuable test, as it is the free T4 that is biologically active.

As discussed earlier, when the brain thinks that the thyroid gland is producing insufficient amounts of the thyroid hormone necessary for action, it has the pituitary gland secrete large amount of thyroid stimulating hormone. If your TSH test is normal and you are still experiencing symptoms related to hypothyroidism, then a free T4 test will help you to diagnose any thyroid related problems. So this test is one of the most trustworthy tests used to diagnose Hashimoto's disorder.

If your test result reveals decreased level of free T4, this means there is thyroid hormone deficiency. This may be possible even if your TSH levels are in normal range.

It is vital that you notice each and every change in your body. The faster you notice any changes, the faster you are diagnosed and the faster and more effective the management of the disease will be, without it doing much damage to the body. This is not just about Hashimoto's disorder. In any case this practice can help you a lot.

So, please do not hesitate to share the details with your doctor and go visit them at the earliest. They will guide you in the most correct and appropriate direction and help you achieve the quickest cure. Remember, hiding anything from your doctor is a harmful practice that can even prove to be a fatal one. Therefore it is necessary to tell your doctor everything and also ask questions even if you feel that it's stupid. When it comes to medical science and your health, no question is stupid.

Estrogen levels

It is very important to check the estrogen levels in the body, because the action of the thyroid hormone produced by the thyroid gland is reduced, if the estrogen levels are higher. Hence you should make it a regular practice to get your hormone levels checked. If they are abnormal, consult a doctor as soon as possible.

Also, blood should be checked for anemia; both iron deficiency and pernicious anemia.

Prognosis

Prognosis is the second step of curing a disease. The prognosis depends on how fast your disease is diagnosed. Thus, if your disease is diagnosed in the very initial stage then the prognosis is good and the quality of prognosis reduces as the patient's health deteriorates. If the diagnosis is not done early and if the condition is left untreated for too long, then the prognosis is too slow and therefore bad. Thus prognosis is solely based upon the time, stage and quality of the diagnosis. Wrong diagnosis can ruin the prognosis and thus can hinder the treatment process or even cause a fiasco.

Veronica Baruwal

Chapter 5

How to Prevent Hashimoto's Thyroiditis?

Until now we have been discussing how the Hashimoto's disease can be diagnosed and what its major symptoms are. But prevention of Hashimoto's disorder is one of the most important topics.

For each disease there exists some kind of preventive measures that can be undertaken to avoid it. Unfortunately in the case of disorders this is not possible, as most of the disorders occur suddenly and are caused due to the malfunctioning of certain organs. Hashimoto's is one such disorder. Research has shown that there is no particular prevention that can save you from this disease. You cannot undertake simple measures to avoid it. Luckily this disease can be cured with proper medical care and treatment. But, like in the case of every disorder and disease, it is cheaper and less time consuming if the problem is diagnosed early. The earlier you are diagnosed with the disease, the faster you can start with the treatment. Early treatment also means easy treatment with less pain and fast results. Hence it is always advised to go through a routine check up with your GP once every six months.

Hashimoto's disorder is an autoimmune disease, and doctors are unable to identify the reason behind why the body's protection mechanism destroys the healthy tissue. As explained earlier, it has been proven that there are no solid causes for this disorder. Although, avoiding the things explained in this chapter can definitely help you to keep yourself healthy and away from Hashimoto's, this is not prevention. At best, it can be deemed as protection with no guaranteed results.

Since there are no known ways to prevent this disease, it is very important for an individual to notice the changes in their body and the signs and symptoms of Hashimoto's disease and report them to a doctor as soon as possible. For this reason it is extremely necessary to study and restudy the chapter dealing with symptoms of these diseases twice or thrice, so you can memorize the symptoms and keep an eye on yourself and your loved ones.

Complications of Hashimoto's thyroiditis

Nothing is simple in life and everything has complications, especially disorders and diseases. Every single disease has its own set of complications that are both similar and different compared to the other diseases and disorders. Complications are common in any disease nowadays but don't be misinformed about them. Complications do not limit themselves to the organ of the body that is affected; rather complications are seen over all in the body, sometimes proving to be more harmful than the disease itself.

In the case of Hashimoto's disease, the symptoms of the disorder are seen all over the body. Why does this happen? Hashimoto's is an endocrinal disease, where there is malfunction in synthesis, production and regulation of the thyroid hormone, and thus the effects are noticed all over the body. The disease also happens due to the malfunction of the immune system, which is a very essential mechanism of the body and is related and connected to every corner of the body. So when this system gets affected it can wreak havoc on your body quite easily.

Now let us have a closer look at some of the complications that may arise due to Hashimoto's disorder.

Goiter

Goiter is one of the most common problems that affects the thyroid gland. Goiter is the bloating and swelling of the thyroid gland. As mentioned above, that is a result of low thyroid hormone production. The pituitary gland secretes large amounts of thyroid stimulating hormone in order to stimulate the thyroid gland. Due to this constant stimulation done by the thyroid stimulating hormone, the thyroid gland starts to produce more thyroid hormone to counter it, resulting in an over production of the thyroid hormone and causing the gland to enlarge in size. Anything over produced is a harmful thing and so is the case with this hormone.

Initially the patient may not notice the enlargement but only starts noticing that something is wrong when it starts growing fast. But in some cases, patients do not notice anything at all until it becomes too big. The goiter appears to be a fleshy ball like structure in the throat. The goiter is generally firm in consistency and irregular in shape. It can be of any shape and size. Some goiters are quite little while some can grow up to an abnormal size. If the goiter is too large in size, it can cause difficulty in swallowing as it may compress the esophagus. Difficulty in breathing may also occur because if it is pressing on to the wind pipe. The patient may feel extremely irritated, dejected and depressed because of the above characteristics.

Cardiac problems

The second major complication that may arise due to the Hashimoto's disorder is cardiac sufferings. People who suffer from Hashimoto's thyroiditis are at a higher risk of developing heart problems and have a higher level of bad cholesterol.

Patients complain of frequent chest pain, but heart failure is not common. But even the chest pain is a very painful and harmful thing and can cause a lot of problems.

Mental disorder

As this disease is closely related to the brain and hormones, it can cause problems in the mental and physical health of a person. Psychological problems are highly common in this disorder. Depression may be noticed in Hashimoto's thyroiditis, especially in long standing cases. Patients who suffer from this disease also complain of a decreased sexual drive. This can result into a lot of complications that can lead to a variety of physical and psychological problems.

Other auto immune disease

Patients who are already suffering from Hashimoto's thyroiditis, which is an autoimmune disease, are more at risk of developing many other autoimmune diseases. In this case, Hashimoto's disease acts as a primary cause for developing other diseases. Here is a comprehensive list of some of the diseases that a person suffering from Hashimoto's may contract:

Addison's disease

A patient suffering from Hashimoto's may contract Addison's disease quite easily. This is an autoimmune disease where the immune system attacks the adrenal glands of the body, which are located just above the kidney. This disease has many symptoms. It is characterized by weight loss, poor appetite, muscle weakness, joint pains(which can often be excruciating), and discoloration of the skin, especially hyper pigmentation where the skin pigments get affected and the skin tone changes or gets patchy.

Type 1 diabetes-

This is another disorder that is highly common in patients suffering from Hashimoto's. It's an autoimmune disorder where the immune system attacks the beta cells of Langerhans, which are present in the pancreas. These beta cells are responsible for producing the insulin in the body. This disease is characterized by dryness of the mouth, increased thirst, increased appetite, increased frequency of urination and skin complaints. This disorder can also prove to be harmful as it works as sort of a gateway to other diseases and disorders.

Graves's disease-

Grave's disease is highly common in the patients suffering from Hashimoto's. It is also commonly known as thyrotoxicosis. It is an autoimmune disorder where the white blood cells attack the thyroid gland. Yes, this disease also affects the thyroid gland, but in the complete opposite way than that of Hashimoto's disorder. In this condition there is over production of the thyroid hormone by the thyroid gland. This disease is characterized by symptoms like weight loss, muscle weakness, complete intolerance to heat, increased sweating, more frequent stools, bulging of eyes and many more symptoms. It is a very severe disorder and one you would want to avoid if at all possible.

Systemic lupus erythomatosus-

This disease is characterized by inflammation in all the organs and systems of the body, majorly affecting the respiratory system and cardiac system. Thus this disease is considered to be quite serious.

Rheumatoid arthritis-

This is an autoimmune disorder. This disease affects the small joints of the body, causing inflammation. It is characterized by painful joints; stiffness of joints noticed in the morning, redness and warmth noticed in the joint area and even joint deformities. Because of the frequent or rather continuous pains in the joints, sufferers may not be able to move properly and can develop severe muscle cramps as well. This disorder hinders a person's private, social as well as professional life as the person simply cannot move without causing themselves a lot of pain.

Pernicious anemia-

Anemia is a disorder that affects blood. This happens because the body does not absorb the vitamin B12 properly. Vitamin B12 is very important for developing the red blood cells in the body and thus due to the low absorption or improper absorption of this vitamin the production of the red blood cells stops or malfunctions resulting in the disorder.

Thrombocytopenic purpura-

In this disease condition too, the blood is affected. There is a decrease in the platelet count and so the blood does not clot. The disease is characterized by easy bruising, excessive bleeding from small cuts, bleeding gums, blood in stool and urine, excessive menstrual flow and fatigue. Thus these are some of the most common disorders that can attack a person who is already suffering from the Hashimoto's disease.

Chapter 6
Hashimoto's Disease and Pregnancy

This disease has a long-standing history with pregnancy. The disorder can cause a lot of problems to those who are pregnant as well as their unborn child. Thus, it becomes highly important to keep a check on your health if you are pregnant. In this chapter I will try to make some points clear about pregnancy and Hashimoto's disease, their relation with each other etc.

it is thought that people who undergo menstruation each month. are at higher risk of developing the disease. menstruation causes the body to go through many changes and this can result in hormonal imbalances. Pregnancy results in rapid and various changes in the body, including hormonal changes which may induce Hashimoto's disorder. When someone is pregnant and is also suffering from Hashimoto's disease, further complications are likely unless they seek immediate treatment. Proper medications and timely treatment, when done all through the nine months of pregnancy, can help you avoid any major difficulties during pregnancy.

During pregnancy, the body goes through many hormonal changes. There is a slight rise in the thyroid hormone during pregnancy as well. This rise is not so much that it produces an enlargement such as goiter. a properly working thyroid gland ensures the proper development of the fetus.

It is highly important for those who are pregnant to keep an eye on their health. They should ensure that they notice all the changes taking place in the body, and if they notice the symptoms of Hashimoto's thyroiditis they need to contact their doctor immediately. even if it turns out to be nothing more than a false alarm, it is better to be safe than to be sorry. Consulting a doctor in this matter is highly beneficial because doctors know more about medical related factors than you. A doctor will serve as guide who can help you and show you how to continue with your pregnancy while suffering from this autoimmune disorder.

The thyroid hormone is necessary for the development of the fetus in the womb, especially in the first three months of pregnancy where the development of the brain and nervous system of the baby takes place. Thus the role of the thyroid hormone can actually shape the baby's future. The baby depends on the thyroid hormone produced in the initial few months of pregnancy because the baby has still not developed its own thyroid gland. The baby's thyroid gland is fully ready and starts to function after 12-14 weeks of pregnancy. But even though the thyroid gland is developed, the fetus still depends on the body for iodine supplements. The thyroid gland needs iodine to produce thyroid hormone. Without iodine, there is a chance that goiter might develop.

It is vital to consume at least 250 micrograms of iodine on a daily basis when pregnant to avoid under activity of thyroid gland. This iodine can be consumed in various ways such as consuming iodine-enriched salt.

Now it is quite important to look at the complications that may arise because of the Hashimoto's disorder.

The most common complications in pregnancy with Hashimoto's thyroiditis are as follows:

- Hypertension during pregnancy.
- Pre term delivery of the baby.
- Decreased birth weight of the baby.
- Neurological problems in the child at birth.
- Post pregnancy hemorrhaging, which may also result in severe shock due to excessive blood loss.
- Miscarriage
- Abruption of the placenta
- Severe anemia

If someone remains unaware that they are suffering from Hashimoto's thyroiditis throughout the term of their pregnancy and is thus not treated properly, the child is at a higher risk of developing birth defects. Sometimes this results in stillbirth. Now let us take a look at what complication may arise in babies due to the Hashimoto's disorder. These babies have many problems like:

- Still birth
- Cleft lip
- Delayed teething
- Swelling of muscles, with weak reflexes
- Intellectual impairment
- Delayed or precocious puberty

It is very important for those at childbearing age that wish to have children to undergo regular thyroid screening. If you are pregnant and also suffering from Hashimoto's disease then you need to see your doctor immediately as early treatment will lower the risks during pregnancy. As said earlier, this disorder is curable and thus you should get treated as soon as you suspect anything is wrong so as to avoid the aforementioned problems.

Is it safe to take thyroid medication during pregnancy?

You may be wondering if the thyroid medication will cause any problems with your pregnancy and your unborn child. In this section I have tried to answer your query.

It is highly important to consult a doctor before starting new medication when pregnant. All you need to do is visit your gynecologist and endocrinologist throughout the nine months of pregnancy and they will guide you in the right directions.

Although everything needs to be done with the permission of the doctor, I have provided the names of some of the most common tablets and medicines that are normally prescribed during such times. It should be noted that these names have been provided just for the purpose of information; this should not be treated as a prescription without seeing your doctor as any medicine or drug that has not been prescribed by a doctor can cause harm to you and your fetus. Now let us have a look at these medicines.

During pregnancy it is safe to ingest levothyroxine. This takes care of the health of the fetus as well. But what you had been taking the medicine before pregnancy? in this case you may be required to increase the dosage of the medicine for normal thyroid functioning.

It is very important to get your thyroid test done every 6-8 weeks during your pregnancy so that if there is any change in the thyroid hormone reading the doctor can help you out and preventing further complications.

The thyroid often starts to function normally again after pregnancy and you can go back to your previous dosage of levothyroxine. So you can once again lead a relatively normal life.

Hashimoto's disease and breast feeding

There are no known issues with breastfeeding when it comes to this disease. Sufferers are still able to breastfeed their babies without any risks.

However, Hashimoto's attacks the thyroid system, which plays an important role in the production of milk. Unfortunately due to this disorder the system malfunctions and thus sufferers may not produce enough or any milk. Treatment is available though to alleviate this problem. Levothyroxine is the best medication to take while breastfeeding. It cannot affect your child's health as not only is it harmless but it cannot pass into the milk produced.

Pregnancy is a delicate time for the body and hence it is important to pay attention to every small change the body goes through to make sure nothing is amiss.

In the next chapter we will look at some of the most common modes of treating the Hashimoto's disorder.

Chapter 7
Treatments for Hashimoto's

Although prevention is better than a cure, in some cases prevention may not be a possibility. Hashimoto's is one such disease for which there are no preventive measures, as previously discussed. It is thus important to concentrate on treatments available for this disorder. In this chapter, I have listed out all the treatments that are available for the Hashimoto's disorder.

If Hashimoto's is diagnosed early, it can be treated in the best possible way. Early diagnosis is important as it can be treated much faster and can cost you a lot less money. There are many treatments available for curing Hashimoto's disorder on the market, but unfortunately many these cannot cure the disorder and will rip you off. Thyroid hormone replacement therapy is the only treatment that is available that will completely cure Hashimoto's thyroiditis.

Thyroid hormone replacement therapy is a treatment which supplies you with that extra thyroid hormone which your body is lacking due to your thyroid gland malfunctioning. The amount of the thyroid hormone you need is reintroduced in your body with the help of various methods. Thyroid hormone replacement therapy is the most effective therapy for treating Hashimoto's thyroiditis.

This therapy might be strange to some people which is why it is important to explain what exactly the thyroid replacement theory is, and how it works.

How does thyroid replacement therapy work?

Many hormones are produced by the thyroid gland, out of which the following two, Triiodothyronine (T3) and tetraiodothyronine (T4), are the two major ones. These are extremely essential hormones and they play a very important role in the day-to-day functioning of the body.

Tetraiodothyronine is the hormone that is provided to you artificially by thyroid replacement therapy. The therapy will only provide you with the T4 hormone because the body converts the T3 hormone into T4 hormone. This is why it is advisable to take only T4 hormone and not take a combination of T3 and T4. T4 hormone stays in the body for a longer period of time. Levothyroxine is the most appropriate T4 hormone type that can be ingested, if directed by a physician. It is considered to be highly safe and effective.

Levothyroxine does not have any major side effects. It may be possible that in the initial days you may experience mild headaches and giddiness, which happens because your body is not used to the influx of the correct amounts of the thyroid hormone. As days pass, you will not experience these symptoms any longer. Your body gets attuned to the therapy very quickly.

Levothyroxine, when taken regularly, helps normalize the thyroid hormone levels in the body. The symptoms of Hashimoto's thyroiditis start to vanish as your hormone level reaches a normal level. You will once again feel healthy and you might also feel that your body and mind are rejuvenated.

Keep a watch on the dose that you are taking

Like every other thing in this world, excess Levothyroxine can be a curse. Remember that the dosage of Levothyroxine that needs to be ingested by the patient depends up on the severity of their symptoms. Each individual is different and they all come up with varied intensity of symptoms, and so the dosage of the doses differs accordingly. The symptoms of the person may seem similar to that of another person, but it is very important to understand that the two patients are two different individuals with strikingly different bodies and one person's medicine should not be used by another person without the advice of a doctor.

The doctor will decide about your medicinal dose. The patient should not interfere with the medicine and should not try to change the dosage at home, no matter what their opinion is or what they may have read elsewhere. Doing so might have disastrous consequences for the patient.

There are patients who try to change their dosage as and when they notice some changes in their health such as when their symptoms start to disappear or lessen in intensity. It is dangerous to do this without your doctor's approval.

If you suspect that you are improving and your dosage should be changed, visit your doctor and consult with them. If you are still uncertain, it would be no harm to seek the opinion of a different doctor too. Sometimes the doctors ask for laboratory investigations and then, based on the thyroid hormone reading, take a decision of changing the dose.

Medicine which interfere with levothyroxine

It is quite possible that your current medicines may interact with Levothyroxine and this may cause problems or complications.

There are many known substances and medications which interfere with the action of Levothyroxine by not allowing the blood to absorb the medicine effectively.

Before starting this hormone replacement therapy, the patient should talk to the doctor about the other medicines that they are taking on regular basis in order to stop any interference from any components in those medicines.

These are a list of few medicines to avoid when taking Levothyroxine-

- Multivitamin tablets, especially the ones which have excess quantities of iron supplement in them

- Antacids, which are used for treating acidity, as they contain aluminum hydroxide, which affects the absorption

- Medicines that are taken for reducing blood cholesterol levels

- Medicines that have high calcium levels

- Medication that are used to treat ulcers and gastrointestinal issues, as these medicines usually contain sucralfate

- Certain antibiotics like ciprofloxacin, norfloxacin, and lomefloxacin.

The aforementioned are just some of the medicines that can cause a lot of complications or may even prevent the absorption of Levothyroxine in your blood stream. It is advisable that you speak to your consulting doctor about all the medicines and supplements that you consume on a regular basis and the impact they may have on your treatment.

Veronica Baruwal

Chapter 8
Hashimoto's Disease and Diet

A disease can be treated quite effectively with medicine but if you want to get cured quickly and effectively, you should always accompany the treatment with a good diet and with regular exercise.

Medication is definitely sufficient for treating Hashimoto's thyroiditis but if you eat correctly and and take your medication, you will recover far sooner.

Things you need to include in your diet

Proteins

Individuals who are suffering from Hashimoto's thyroiditis are advised to consume large amounts of proteins. They should consume a minimum of 20-30 grams of protein with every meal. This means that they should consume 60-90 grams of protein per day on an average. It is better for these patients to consume animal protein like eggs, chicken and fish. Red meats, like beef, should be avoided. If you are a vegetarian, then opt for food like nuts, soya milk, flax seeds and Tempeh. Also try to snack on food products that have good protein value, like roasted almonds or a peanut butter and jelly sandwich. You can also get high amounts of proteins from pulses, sprouts, legumes, etc. Sprouts contain high amounts of proteins and are beneficial for your health. You can also talk to your doctor and take his advice whether you can consume some kind of protein supplement that might help you with this.

Fats

Who says that being and eating healthy means that you should completely avoid fats? This is common myth that keeps on cropping up everywhere. Fat is not a bad thing. Fat is also essential for the body but it is important to include good fats in the diet rather than bad fats, which have no nutritional value. Include fats like olive oil, ghee, coconut oil, chia seeds and flax seeds. Avocados are also a good source of good fats to keep your body healthy.

Anti oxidants

Increase the intake of food products which contain anti oxidants in them. Anti oxidants help the body fight inflammation that is caused by the immune system attacking the body's cell, producing a lot of fire in the thyroid gland.

There are many natural and healthy options available in the market that are full of anti oxidants. You can easily find them in any store.

Green tea is rich in anti oxidants and should be consumed at least three times a day. It should serve as a replacement to your caffeinated beverages. It is one of the best ways to stay healthy. You can find green tea almost everywhere and in many flavors.

Prunes, walnuts, yogurt and black berries are also rich in anti oxidants. Try including them in small amounts between snacks to get nutrition from every meal you consume. Instead of filling your body with junk food, opt for fruit as it is good for your body and can provide you with much needed nutrients without empty calories.

Vegetables

Include fresh vegetables in your diet every day. Choose a large variety of colorful vegetables and include them in your daily meals. You can consume them either by cooking them or you can even enjoy a freshly chopped salad of raw vegetables seasoned with some salt, pepper and vinegar. According to ancient Indian traditions, it is advisable that your plate look as colorful as possible.

Although vegetables are healthy in nearly every form, it should be noted that boiled and raw vegetables are best. Fruit and vegetables that can be eaten raw should always be eaten raw as they are not only full of nutrients but they also promote digestion and are good for your dental health.

Avoid vegetables that belong to brassica family as they can interfere with the functioning of the thyroid gland. These include cauliflower, broccoli and turnips. Try to consume as little of these vegetables as possible.

Water

Drink large quantities of water every day. An individual should consume at least 2-3 liters of water per day. Make sure that the water that you consume is free from chlorine and fluoride as they hamper the thyroid gland functions.

According to one theory, you need to consume one liter of water per 20 kg of your body weight, every day. So, for instance, if your body weight is 60 kg, then you should drink at least 3 liters of water every day.

If you do not feel like drinking water all the time you can add some lemon to the water or you can add lemon and honey to make a tasty drink that you will surely gulp down.

However, drinking too much water can cause more harm than good. This is why most health experts recommend that you only drink when you are thirsty and should not force yourself to drink water otherwise just to fill a daily quota. However, most people will drink the healthy amount of water for their body every day simply by drinking when they're thirsty, providing they avoid caffeinated beverages and alcohol.

Carbohydrates

One should also include carbohydrates in their diet. Include whole grains, pulses, and cereals. People who suffer from Hashimoto's thyroiditis also have problems with digestion and have a slow metabolism. Pulses are best digested when they are soaked overnight, so pre prep them rather than consuming them on a whim.

Also, you should make sure to chew your food properly as this aids in improving digestion. If a person does not chew properly or eats too quickly, they may suffer from problems such as constipation, IBS etc.

Vitamins

Vitamins are some of the most essential nutrients that help keep our body going. All vitamins should be consumed in their prescribed quantities in order for the body to use them effectively.

<u>Vitamin A</u>- food like carrots, yogurt, spinach, red bell peppers, and squash

Vitamin C- food products like lime, fruits rich in citric acid, and parsley.

Minerals

Iodine deficiency is one of the major causes of developing Hashimoto's thyroiditis. Iodine is the most essential mineral in order for the thyroid gland to function properly. Choose iodized salt instead of table salt, because extra iodine is mixed in iodized salt. Seafood and seaweeds are a good source of iodine. Apparently some types of mountain salt have iodine but these can be rare to find. Thus it, is advised to use the iodized salt that is commonly and easily available in the market.

Selenium - Selenium deficiency is also one of the causes of this disorder. Consume oats, sunflower seeds, shrimp, Brazil nuts, and brown rice as they are rich in selenium. However, selenium has been the source of much medical controversy lately so it will be better if you consult your doctor or GP before you up the quantities of selenium you consume.

Food products that you need to avoid

There are certain foods products that you need to avoid if you are suffering from this autoimmune disease. These food products can actually increase the severity of the disorder or may cause complications. Following is a short list of products that you must avoid.

- Most sources of gluten
- Unsaturated oil
- Soy
- Processed foods

Chapter 9
Paleolithic Diet and Recipes

There is popular notion that the Paleo diet can help people suffering from this disorder and any other form of autoimmune diseases. Although this claim is not scientifically proven yet, I am including a short introduction to the Paleo diet and also including some of the most delicious and healthy recipes that can help you cure this disorder. Even if it doesn't cure you, it will keep you healthy.

But, before heading to the recipes section, it is necessary to understand what the Paleo diet exactly is.

Paleo diet is basically a diet that is based upon the dietary habits and practices of those in the Stone Age or Paleolithic era. So, in this diet the you are supposed to eat and drink what our ancestors used to. Therefore, a person who is following this diet simply cannot consume anything that has been processed or eat things that were not consumed by our ancestors.

People are now aware that what they eat has consequences on their body, and what a certain diet can do for our bodies, both positively and negatively. Our lifestyle can also induce problems such as obesity, diabetes as well as cardiovascular diseases.

The aforementioned diseases are becoming increasingly common nowadays due to the fact that our lifestyle is changing rapidly and we tend to lead a sedentary way of life. Due to this, our dietary habits too are changing, but unfortunately our genes are not. Our genetic makeup is still nearly the same as that as of our ancestors- the cavemen. Our diets have changed much faster than our bodies can handle.

Thus, it is wise that a lot of people are now moving towards and choosing the Paleo diet. This diet is better as compared to other diets, as it is not only a good diet to lose weight, but it can also help you control your auto immune disorders as well. *

This diet is also revolutionary as it calls for a total abstinence from processed foods, which is hard in this day and age. You can also effectively cut your levels of carbohydrates with this diet. The carbs derived from refined sugars and grains are bad for your health and this diet helps you to stay away from them.

The people who follow this diet consume a high amount of proteins that they get from seafood and lean meats. They also eat foods rich with vitamins and minerals thanks to the large amount of fruits and vegetables that they consume. These nutrients keep you healthy and fit and also boost your immune system which is vital for this disorder.

But it is necessary to understand that only following the Paleo diet is not enough. You also need to do physical activities, such as exercising regularly, and you need to get enough sleep as well. This ensures that your body remains fit and healthy.

Veronica Baruwal

Now let us go forward and have a look at some of the most common recipes that you can enjoy while following the Paleo diet. These recipes are quite easy to prepare and extremely delectable to taste. These recipes are also full of nutrients and are highly beneficial for your health.

Tangy Orange Bread with Poppy Seeds

Serves: 4

Ingredients

- 3 ½ tbsp homemade orange jam (sugar free)
- ½ cup of each sunflower butter, tahini and almond butter – mixed
- 6 eggs
- 2 tsp orange essence
- 1 ½ tsp cider vinegar
- ¾ cup tapioca flour
- 1 ½ tsp ground vanilla
- 3 tbsp poppy seeds
- 3 tbsp ground chia seeds
- ¾ tsp salt
- 1 ½ tsp baking soda

Preparation

1. Keep the oven on preheat mode at 350 F.

2. In a bowl mix the butters, vinegar, jam, eggs and essence.

3. In another bowl mix salt, soda and flour. Now add the seeds to this bowl.

4. Slowly fold the content of the second bowl into the first one.

5. Pour into a greased tray and the place it in the oven. Bake for 30 to 40 minutes.

6. Remove from oven and cool for 10 minutes before inverting on a wire rack.

7. Serve with some homemade strawberry jam or a dash of honey.

La Piperade

<u>Serves: 3</u>

<u>Ingredients</u>

- 2.5 tbsp olive oil
- 5 green bell peppers, cut into small pieces
- 1.5 cup bacon, diced
- 3 onions, chopped
- 5 tomatoes, peeled
- 2.5 cloves of garlic, chopped
- 5 eggs beaten
- Salt and pepper to taste

<u>Preparation</u>

1. Heat some oil in a pan.
2. Add the peppers, bacon and the onion and sauté till the onions become soft.

3. Next, add tomatoes and crush them using a crusher or a masher. Next, add the seasonings and the garlic.

4. Finally add the eggs and let it cook.

5. Scramble the eggs.

6. Serve immediately.

Crepes

Serves: 3

Ingredients

- 3 eggs
- ½ cup water
- ¼ cup arrowroot powder
- Salt
- 2 tsp coconut oil for greasing

Preparation

1. In a bowl add all the ingredients, except the coconut oil and whisk to create a loose batter.
2. Grease a pan and preheat it on a medium flame.
3. Pour some of the batter on the pan spread it in the bottom of the pan by swirling the pan around.
4. Let the crepe cook for a bit, flip and cook till it is golden brown.

5. Repeat with the remaining batter and serve with a side of strawberries.

Apricot Pesto Chicken with Basil

Serves: 4

Ingredients

- ½ cup dried apricots, halved
- 1 tsp almond flour
- 2 lb. chicken breasts, skinless and boneless
- 1 cup fresh basil leaves
- 1 garlic clove, minced
- 2 tbsp olive oil
- ½ fresh lemon, juices
- Pinch of salt and pepper

Preparation

1. Keep the oven on preheat mode at 350 degree F.
2. In a food processor, blend the flour and apricots to get a paste like consistency. Keep this aside.

3. In a bowl mix all the ingredients except chicken and blend using an electronic beater.

4. Mix this blended concoction with the almond paste.

5. Slice the chicken breast horizontally to create a pocket.

6. Stuff the filling we have prepared in this pocket and then bake the breast in the preheated oven for 30 minutes.

7. Remove the breast from the oven and then put on the remaining paste on the chicken. Once again bake of 10 minutes.

8. Remove from oven and allow to cool for a few minutes before serving.

Potato Salad Packing with Probiotics

Serves: 2 to 3

Ingredients

- 4 to 5 red skinned potatoes.

- 4 to 5 strips of Bacon

- 1/4 cup of chopped sauerkraut (Ensure that it is fermented by lacto sources and not vinegar)

- 1/4 cup of chopped spring onions

- 2 tablespoons of mustard sauce

- 2 or 3 tablespoons of organic apple cider vinegar

- 2/4 cup of mayo (use vegan mayo if you are a vegetarian or a vegan)

- Salt to taste

Preparation

1. Ensure that your oven has been preheated to about 345-350F.

2. Boil the potatoes and do not peel them in salted water for about half an hour or until they become soft.

3. Drain the potatoes and dice them into smaller bits after they are boiled.

4. Bake the strips of bacon for about 40 minutes until they turn crispy and golden.

5. Once all of it is set combine the potatoes and the strips of bacon in a large bowl and add in the chopped sauerkraut and chopped spring onions.

6. Combine mayo, apple cider vinegar and mustard sauce and mix them together with salt.

7. Pour this dressing over the salad and give the salad a toss.

Avocado Cucumber Summer Cold Soup

Serves: 4 to 6

Ingredients

- 3 large Persian cucumbers (you can also use regular cucumbers if you want)
- 2 ripe chopped avocados
- ½ cup of chopped fresh mint leaves
- Juice of 1-2 lemons
- 1/2 cup of fresh chopped coriander
- 5-6 peeled and chopped almonds
- 1 tablespoon of lemon zest
- Salt to taste
- 1-2 tablespoons of extra virgin olive oil
- 2 cloves of chopped garlic
- 2 tablespoons cumin

Preparation

1. Chop the cucumber into quarters. You don't need to peel the cucumbers.

2. Peel and chop some avocados.

3. Take a pan and add the cumin to this and let it toast for about a minute or until you can smell the cumin aroma.

4. Take the toasted cumin and grind it coarsely using a pestle and mortar.

5. Combine the juice of 1-2 lemons and lemon zest along with the cumin and salt.

6. Add this mixture to the garlic, cucumber and avocados into a blender along with the mint and coriander and blend till it is a smooth paste like consistency.

7. Put the soup into the fridge or you can add ice cubes if you want.

8. Add some olive oil over the top and add the almonds to this soup.

Almond Bread

Serves: 4 to 6 1 loaf with about 12 slices

Ingredients

- 1 and half tablespoons of toasted flax seed
- 1 tablespoons of apple cider vinegar
- 4 to 5 tablespoons water
- 1 tablespoons of organic honey
- 1 tablespoons coconut oil
- 1 teaspoon of baking soda
- 1/3 cups of almond flour
- 4 tablespoons of chopped almonds
- Salt to taste

Preparation

1. Ensure that the oven has been preheated to about 300 degrees F.

2. Ground the toasted flax seeds with a pestle and mortar and add water to this mixture. Leave the mixture to sit for a while and this will form a gel.

3. Take a bowl and add the almond flour along with the baking soda, salt and chopped almonds.

4. Take the flaxseed gel and add honey and apple cider vinegar along with coconut oil and mix this.

5. Mix the wet and dry ingredients together and ensure no lumps are formed.

6. Take a baking tray and grease it using a little bit of coconut oil.

7. Pour the mixture into the baking tray and let it bake for about 30 to 40 minutes or until the knife inserted comes out clean.

Dill, Asparagus, and Fennel Soup

Serves: 4

Ingredients

- 6 to 7 snap peas
- 3 large fennel bulbs
- 3-4 asparagus
- 1 tablespoon of lemon zest
- 1/2 cup fresh chopped mint leaves
- ½ cup of spring onions
- Salt to taste
- 2 large leeks
- 2 tablespoons of olive oil
- 1/2 cups of chopped fresh dill
- 3-4 cups of vegetable broth
- 2-3 tablespoons of fresh lemon juice

- 1 tablespoon of crushed black pepper

<u>Preparation</u>

1. After stringing the snap peas ensure you chop them coarsely.

2. Cut the fennel bulbs and ensure it comes to about 2 cups.

3. Cut the asparagus into little bits.

4. Heat water in a pan and add salt and all the vegetables.

5. Put a lid on top of the pot and let it simmer for about 20 to 30 minutes.

6. Take the spring onions and chop them.

7. Fry them with a little bit of olive oil and add some salt and pepper.

8. Cook them until they turn translucent or golden in color.

9. Add the onions and the mint leaves along with the dill leaves to the vegetable broth that has been simmering.

10. Let it come to another boil to incorporate the fresh herb flavor.

11. Add pepper at this point.

12. Let the broth cool for a little while and then add them in a blender.

13. Blend the broth until it becomes a soupy consistency.

14. Add more salt, pepper and add the lemon juice and lemon zest and stir.

15. Boil one last time.

16. Add a little bit of olive oil and serve hot.

Apple and Zucchini Pancakes Made with Almond Flour

Serves: 5 to 6 pancakes

Ingredients

- 1 cup of grated zucchini
- 2 tablespoons of coconut oil
- 4-5 tablespoons of chopped fresh thyme
- 2/3 cup of grated apple
- 1 cup almond flour
- 1 tablespoon organic honey, you an also use maple syrup instead
- 1/2 teaspoon baking powder
- Salt to taste
- 1 knob or 2 tablespoons of almond butter or any other nut butter
- 3 eggs

Preparation

1. Add the grated zucchini and grated apple in a bowl.
2. Heat a pan and add the knob of butter and add the thyme to it.
3. Let it sit for about 10 seconds and then add it to the zucchini and apple mixture. Add honey to this.
4. Add the almond flour along with some salt and baking powder in another bowl.
5. Break three eggs and beat the eggs slightly.
6. Combine all ingredients together.
7. Pour coconut oil in a pan and pour the pancake batter.
8. Let each side cook for 3-4 minutes.
9. Serve hot.

Veronica Baruwal

Quinoa with Nuts and Goji Berries

<u>Serves: 4</u>

<u>Ingredients</u>

- 1 cup of quinoa, you can use white or red quinoa.
- 2 cups of water
- 1/3 tablespoon of basil
- 1/3 tablespoon of coriander
- 1 teaspoon of cumin seeds
- 1/3 tablespoon of parsley
- 1/3 cup of Goji berries
- 1/3 cup of mixed nuts (almonds, cashews, pistachios, walnuts)
- Salt or sugar to taste

<u>Preparation</u>

1. Soak the quinoa grains for 5 to 10 minutes in a bowl.

2. Soak the Goji berries in another bowl with warm water for 5 to 10 minutes.

3. Drain the quinoa and put it in a pot of hot boiling water and cook till it becomes soft or for about 15 minutes.

4. Take the cumin seeds and toast them on a pan and then grind them coarsely with a pestle and mortal.

5. Add the Goji berries along with the cumin seeds and salt or sugar into the quinoa.

6. Add the basil, coriander and parsley.

7. Serve hot.

Veronica Baruwal

Celery root and Squash Soup

Serves: 4 to 5

Ingredients

- 1kg kabocha squash (you can use regular squash if you want).
- 1 large celery root
- 2 tablespoons coconut oil,
- Salt to taste
- 2 leeks
- 1 large onion
- 2-3 tablespoons of chopped sage
- 2-3 tablespoons of chopped rosemary
- 2 cups of vegetable stock
- Juice of 1 lemon
- 1 tablespoon of lemon zest
- 1 tablespoon of pepper

- ½ teaspoon of chili flakes
- 2 spoon any nut butter
- Pumpkin seeds

Preparation

1. Peel the squash and dice it into cubes.

2. Chop the celery into bits.

3. Put the two chopped vegetables in a pot of water. Let it simmer for half an hour or until they become very soft. Alternatively you can pressure cook them.

4. Take a pan and pour the coconut oil in it, once the oil is hot add the slices of onions and fry them till they turn translucent or golden brown. Chop the leaks and add the chopped leaks to this and fry them as well.

5. Drain the celery and squash.

6. Add the vegetable stock along with the rosemary and sage to the cooked vegetables. Also add the onion and leaks.

7. Let the broth cook for about 20 minutes or so.

8. Add the knobs of butter, chili flakes and lemon juice along with the zest of one lemon.

9. After the mixture is cooked, let it cool for a while.

10. Blend this mixture till it forms a soup like consistency.

11. Add pepper and salt at this point and stir well.

12. Give it another boil and add pumpkin seeds

13. Serve hot.

Raw Marinated Mushrooms

Serves: 8

Ingredients

- 4 lb thinly sliced white mushrooms
- 8 tbsp apple cider vinegar
- Freshly ground black pepper
- Chopped cilantro
- 12 tbsp of olive oil, cold pressed
- 2 tsp each of salt and dried rosemary, sage and thyme

Preparation

1. In a bowl add the oil, vinegar, salt, pepper and the herbs. Mix well.
2. Toss in the mushrooms and let them marinate for 10 minutes.
3. Serve garnished with cilantro.

Veronica Baruwal

Warm Oysters with Vinaigrette

Serves: 4

Ingredients

- 4 dozen oysters
- 2 cup vinegar
- 1 tbsp fresh chives, minced
- 4 tomatoes, peeled and minced
- 2 shallot, minced
- 1 tsp pepper
- Salt, to taste

Preparation

1. Keep the oven on preheat mode at 500 degree F.
2. Take a baking dish and line it with salt. Heat this dish in oven for 15 minutes.
3. In a bowl add the tomatoes, vinegar, shallots, pepper and salt. Mix well and keep aside.

4. Cook the oysters by placing them in the salt lined dish. Bake them for 8 minutes at least.

5. Take them out of the oven and let them cool. Now, cut the muscle that holds the two shells together.

6. While serving remove the upper shell and put it on a plate. Add the vinaigrette to this and serve immediately.

Veronica Baruwal

Grill Zucchini Hummus

<u>Serves: 4</u>

<u>Ingredients</u>

- 2 zucchinis, sliced lengthwise
- 4 cloves of garlic, chopped and crushed
- 1 tbsp fresh basil, chopped
- 1 tsp dried oregano
- 1 tsp fresh parsley, chopped
- 1 tbsp fresh lemon juice
- 1/2 cup sesame seed butter
- Pinch of salt and ground cayenne pepper
- Coconut oil

<u>Preparation</u>

1. Preheat a grill and grease it lightly with oil.
2. Grill the zucchini on the grill till it become tender on both the sides. Keep aside.

3. In a blender add all the ingredients, except parsley. Blend for a few seconds.

4. Add the zucchini and blend till done. The texture should become smooth.

5. Serve with a side of chips.

Veronica Baruwal

Apricot Power Bars

<u>Serves: 6</u>

<u>Ingredients</u>

- 4 cups dried apricots
- 7 cups pecans
- 3 tbsp vanilla extract
- 6 eggs
- Sea salt

<u>Preparation</u>

1. Keep the oven on preheat mode at 325 degree F.
2. In a blender add apricot and pecans and blend till a gravel like texture is achieved.
3. Add the remaining ingredients and blend once again.
4. Put this mixture in a greased baking tray.
5. Bake for 30 minutes or till the mixture is firm to touch.

6. Cool completely before removing from tray. Cut into bars and serve.

Veronica Baruwal

Egg Muffins Delight

Serves: 5

Ingredients

- 12 eggs
- ½ cup tomatoes, chopped
- 1 cup fresh basil, chopped
- Coconut oil
- Salt and pepper to taste

Preparation

1. Keep the oven on preheat mode at 350 degrees.
2. Add some eggs, salt and pepper in a bowl and whisk thoroughly.
3. Now add the tomatoes and basil. Mix well to combine.
4. Grease a muffin tray or muffin tins and pour the prepared batter in them.
5. Bake for 20-25 minutes or till done.

6. You can also add other vegetable according to your taste and choice.

7. Serve hot!

Delicious Breakfast Hash

Serves: 4

Ingredients

- 5 tbsp coconut oil
- 2 onions, sliced thinly
- Pepper, to taste
- 2 tsp dried oregano
- 2 apple, chopped into cubes
- 3 cups Brussels sprouts, chopped finely
- 5 fried eggs
- 5 bacon slices, cooked and minced

Preparation

1. Heat some oil in a skillet and cook onions in it till done.
2. Add the oregano and pepper to this and sauté till aromatic.

3. Add the apples to the pan and once again cook till the apples are tender, yet firm.

4. Add Brussels sprout to the skillet and cook till they are soft.

5. Finally add the eggs and bacon and cook until they are completely cooked.

6. Serve hot.

Veronica Baruwal

Fruit and chicken salad

<u>Serves: 3</u>

<u>Ingredients</u>

- 1 lb chicken breast
- 1/2 cup cranberries (dried)
- 1 apple, peeled and diced
- 1 avocado, peeled and cut
- 1 cup green grapes, cut in half
- 1/2 cup Paleo mayonnaise
- 1 tsp lemon juice
- Salt and pepper to taste

<u>Preparation</u>

1. Cook the chicken according to your taste and then slice it finely. It can be a simple roast, or you can even use leftover chicken from before.
2. Take a bowl and add lemon juice, mayonnaise and salt and pepper to it. Mix well.

3. Take another bowl and mix all the remaining ingredients together.

4. Just before serving, combine the contents of the two bowls together and serve immediately.

Veronica Baruwal

Delicious Pepper Chicken Stir-fry

Serves: 6

Ingredients

- 3 tbsp coconut oil
- 3 tbsp coconut amino
- 6 cooked chicken breasts
- 6 cut bell peppers
- 1 tsp chili powder
- Salt and pepper according to taste

Preparation

1. In a frying pan heat some oil on medium heat.
2. Sauté the bell peppers until tender.
3. Add the chicken, coconut aminos and chili powder.
4. Next add salt and pepper.
5. Cook till the chicken is done.
6. Serve hot.

Tuna Avocado Wraps in Lettuce

<u>Serves: 6</u>

<u>Ingredients</u>

- 3 cans tuna
- 7 large lettuce leaves
- 3 scallions, diced
- 7 tbsp green chilies, diced
- 7 tbsp Paleo mayonnaise
- 1 cup green olives cut in half
- 2 ripe avocado

<u>Preparation</u>

1. Blend the avocado in a blender till a smooth paste is formed.
2. Add the mayonnaise to this. And blend to form a smooth paste.
3. In a bowl add this mixture, chilies, scallions and tuna. Also add the olives.

4. Place a lettuce leaf on a flat surface and spoon some of the mixture on this leaf and wrap the leaf around it. Repeat with the rest of the lettuce leaves.

5. Serve with a side of your favorite Paleo friendly sauce.

Baked Salmon in Maple Syrup

<u>Serves: 3</u>

<u>Ingredients</u>

- ½ lb salmon
- 2 tbsp maple syrup
- 2 garlic clove, minced
- 2 tbsp parsley, chopped
- 2 tbsp coconut aminos
- Pinch of garlic powder, salt and pepper

<u>Preparation</u>

1. Take a mixing bowl and mix all the ingredients except the salmon.
2. Place the salmon in a dish and pour the above mixture over it. Do not rub the marinade into the fish.
3. Marinate for at least an hour.
4. Keep an oven on preheat mode at 400 degree F.

5. Take a pan and grease it lightly.

6. Put the salmon mixture on this pan and cook without cover for 20 minutes or till it is done.

7. Serve hot.

Southwest Omelets

Serves: 7

Ingredients

- 14 eggs, beaten
- Salt and pepper according to taste
- 5 tsp coconut oil
- 3 cups spinach
- 2 yellow onion, diced
- 3 tomatoes, diced
- 3 bell peppers, diced
- 1 lb cooked ham, diced

Preparation

1. Heat a skillet and grease it with coconut oil.
2. In a bowl mix all the ingredients except the vegetables and meat.

3. Pour a quarter of the aforementioned mixture into the preheated and pre greased pan and spread it lightly.

4. On one half of the egg add a little of meat and vegetables.

5. Let it cook.

6. Fold the other half over this and cook till done.

7. Repeat with the remaining batter.

8. Serve hot!

Sweet Potato Hash

Serves: 6

Ingredients

- 3 sweet potatoes, shredded
- 6 egg whites
- 3 tbsp cinnamon
- Salt
- Coconut oil

Preparation

1. In a bowl add sweet potatoes, cinnamon and egg whites. The potatoes should get coated with the egg.
2. Take a skillet and heat some oil in it.
3. Pour a tablespoon of the prepared mixture into the skillet.
4. Flatten the mixture.
5. Fry till brown from both the sides.

6. Repeat with the remaining mixture.

7. Serve hot!

Chocolate Doughnuts with Coffee

Serves: 8

Ingredients

- 4 bananas
- 1 cup coconut flour
- 7 dates, pitted
- 2 tsp vanilla extract
- 1 tsp cinnamon
- 1/2 cup honey
- 4 eggs
- Pinch of salt
- 3 tbsp coconut oil
- Pinch of baking soda and baking powder
- 1 cup dark chocolate chips, melted
- 2 tsp ground coffee

Preparation

1. Keep the oven on preheat mode at 375 degree F.

2. In a food processor, add the honey, dates and bananas and blend till it forms a smooth paste.

3. Add eggs, flour, vanilla, oil, cinnamon, soda, baking powder and salt to the blender jar and blend once again.

4. Grease a doughnut pan and pour the mixture in it.

5. Bake for 20-25 minutes or till thoroughly done.

6. Let it cool.

7. Meanwhile melt some chocolate on a double boiler. Add the coffee to the chocolate.

8. Dip the doughnut in the chocolate and serve.

Turkey Salad with Avocado and Lettuce

Serves: 4

Ingredients

- 8 tbsp olive oil
- 4 avocados, halved
- 4 red bell peppers, diced
- 2 lb turkey, cooked and diced
- 4 cups jicama, peeled and diced
- 2 cup fresh cilantro, chopped
- 6 tsp chili-garlic sauce
- 4 cups red onions, diced
- 6 tbsp fresh lime juice
- Salt and pepper according to taste
- Romaine lettuce leaves

Preparation

1. In a blender blend olive oil, avocado, lime juice and sauce till a thick paste is formed.

2. Add salt and pepper to the prepared paste.

3. Take a bowl and add the onions, turkey, pepper, jicama and some of the cilantro.

4. Toss well to combine.

5. Add the avocado mixture to the bowl.

6. Toss well to coat.

7. For serving, use the lettuce leaves as a base and then spoon the salad on the lettuce leaf.

8. Garnish with cilantro and serve.

Easy Pan Chicken With Green Peas and Butternut Squash

Serves: 8

Ingredients

- 4 cups cooked chicken, minced
- 1/2 cup coconut cream
- 4 tbsp apple cider vinegar
- 1/2 cup green peas, thawed
- 3 tsp seasoning salt
- 3 cups cooked butternut squash, mashed

Preparation

1. Take a saucepan and heat it over medium heat.
2. Place all the ingredients in the saucepan and mix well.
3. Cook until the chicken is done, stirring occasionally to ensure that the ingredients are not sticking to the bottom of the pan.
4. Serve hot.

Veronica Baruwal

Zesty Salmon with Parsley and Dill

Serves: 4

Ingredients

- 6 oz salmon fillets, rinsed
- 1/2 cup of dry white wine
- 1 onion, chopped
- 2 tbsp dill, chopped
- 1 leek, sliced
- 2 tbsp fresh parsley, chopped
- 6 tablespoons extra virgin olive oil
- 1/2 lemon, juiced
- Salt and pepper according to taste

Preparation

1. Keep the oven on preheat mode at 400 degree F.
2. Marinate the salmon in the wine for around 30 minutes in a fridge.

3. In a bowl add lemon juice, pepper, salt and herbs. Mix well.

4. Cook onions and leek in a skillet till done.

5. Now place the strips of salmon on the pan one by one.

6. Pour the mixture of the onions over this. Add some wine if you want to.

7. Now pour the lemon juice and herbs mixture over this.

8. Bake for around ten minutes or till thoroughly done.

9. Serve hot!

Delicious Cornbread Muffins

Serves: 6

Ingredients

- 1 cup coconut flour
- 7 eggs
- 4 tbsp apple butter
- 1 tsp baking soda
- 2 tbsp honey
- 1 cup coconut oil
- 2 tsp apple cider vinegar

Preparation

1. Keep the oven on preheat mode at 350 degree F.
2. In a bowl add the flour and oil. Mix well to combine.
3. Next, add the eggs and beat the mixture thoroughly. Finally add all the other ingredients.
4. Mix well.

5. Take a muffin pan and grease it well with some oil or a cooking spray.

6. Pour this mixture in the muffin pan and bake for around 20 minutes or till a skewer poked in the center of a muffin comes out clean.

7. Remove the muffin tray from the oven and allow to cool for about 10 minutes before removing the muffins from the mold.

8. These muffins taste delicious, whether served hot or cold!

Fried Okra in Pork Batter

Serves: 2

Ingredients

- ½ cup pork rinds
- ½ cup almond flour
- 2 tbsp water
- 2 egg
- ½ tsp chili powder
- 1 stick grass-fed butter
- 2 cup fresh okra, sliced
- ½ tsp coriander
- Salt
- Seasoning salt

Preparation

1. Take a bowl and add water and eggs. Whisk well to combine and make a frothy mixture.

2. Grind the pork till a fine texture is achieved. Mix in the seasoning and the almond flour to this.

3. Take the okra and dip it in the egg mixture and then in the pork batter.

4. Heat some butter in a skillet over a medium flame.

5. Add the okra to this skillet and fry till golden brown from all the sides.

6. Use a napkin or kitchen towel to soak up excess grease and serve hot.

Grilled Steak

Serves: 7

Ingredients

- 3 lb flank steak
- 3 cloves garlic, peeled
- 2 tbsp coconut amino
- 1/2 cup vinegar
- 1/2 cup fresh cilantro
- 1 tbsp fish sauce
- 1 shallot, peeled and halved
- 1/2 cup olive oil
- Pepper
- Salt

Preparation

1. In a blender add everything except the steak and prepare a puree. The puree doesn't need to be very smooth and can contain some lumps.

2. Marinate the steaks in this puree for 6 hours in a fridge or if feasible, overnight.

3. Turn the steaks over in the marinade every few hours to ensure proper marinating.

4. Preheat a grill and then grill the steaks for about 10 minutes on each side for a medium rare steak. You can adjust the timing of cooking as per your preference.

5. Serve hot with a side of some mashed sweet potatoes or grilled vegetables.

Sausage and Asparagus Casserole

Serves: 5

Ingredients

- Coconut oil
- 2 pound sausage, cut
- 14 eggs, whisked
- 1/2 tsp garlic powder
- 8 stalks of asparagus, chopped
- 1/2 cup coconut milk
- 1 leek, sliced
- 1 tbsp fresh dill, minced
- Salt and pepper according to taste

Preparation

1. Keep the oven on preheat mode at 325 degree F.
2. Take a skillet and heat it lightly. Add sausages to the pan sauté them.

3. When half done add the leek and the asparagus. Cook till sausage is cooked through and the leek and asparagus are tender, yet firm.

4. In a bowl add eggs, garlic powder, milk, salt, dill and pepper. Whisk well to form a light and frothy mix.

5. Combine the egg mixture with the sausages and mix well.

6. Take an oven safe pan and grease it well using some coconut oil.

7. Pour the prepared batter in the pan and bake it for 40 minutes or till done.

8. Serve hot.

Delicious Tomato and Dill Frittata

Serves: 10-12

Ingredients

- 9 tomatoes, diced
- 18 eggs, whisked
- 5 garlic cloves, minced
- 5 tbsp fresh dill, chopped
- 2 tsp red pepper flakes
- 5 tbsp fresh chives, chopped
- Coconut oil
- Salt and pepper according to taste

Preparation

1. Keep the oven on preheat mode at 325 degree F.
2. In a bowl mix together the tomatoes, eggs, cloves, dill, red pepper and chives. Season with salt and pepper according to taste.

3. Take an oven safe pan and grease it with the coconut oil.

4. Pour some of the batter in the pan and spread it in the bottom of the pan by swirling the pan around. It should form an inch thick layer.

5. Bake it for around 30 minutes or till done.

6. Do the same for the remaining batter.

7. Serve hot!

Prosciutto Peach Salad with an Arugula Dressing

Serves: 4

Ingredients

- 2 ripe peaches cut into 12 slices
- 12 thin slices of prosciutto
- 2 tbsp almonds, slivered
- 2 tbsp olive oil
- 5 cups baby arugula
- 1 tbsp vinegar
- Salt and pepper according to taste

Preparation

1. Take a slice of prosciutto and roll it on a slice of peach. Repeat with all the slices of prosciutto and pear.
2. Preheat an oven for three minutes at 350 degrees F and then grill prosciutto wrapped pear slices for 3 minutes or more. The meat should become crisp.

3. In a mixing bowl add oil, salt, vinegar, pepper and arugula. Whisk well to combine.

4. Spoon about a tablespoon of the prepared dressing on a plate and place the grilled prosciutto wrapped pear slices in the center. Spoon in some more dressing if you please.

5. Serve immediately.

Chicken Enchilada Bake

Serves: 5

Ingredients

- 1 lb cooked chicken, shredded
- 5 green chilies, diced
- 2 garlic clove, minced
- 1 red bell pepper, diced
- 12 oz. enchilada sauce
- 1/2 tsp of chili powder and dried oregano, mixed together
- Salt and pepper to taste
- 4 eggs, whisked
- Cilantro
- Coconut oil

Preparation

1. Keep the oven on preheat mode at 350 degrees F.

2. In a bowl add the enchilada sauce, bell pepper, chilies, chicken, garlic, chili powder and oregano mix, pepper, and salt. Mix well to coat the chicken and bell peppers with the sauce. To ensure that there are no lumps of the seasonings, add the seasonings to the enchilada sauce and dissolve them before pouring the seasoned enchilada sauce onto the other ingredients.

3. Now add eggs and mix once again.

4. Pour this mixture into a greased baking tray and bake in the preheated oven for an hour.

5. Bake for extra fifteen minutes if not done.

6. Let it cool for 5 minutes and then serve immediately, topped with some cilantro.

Sausage Frittata

Serves: 4

Ingredients

- 3 tbsp coconut oil
- 1 pound Italian sausage, crumbled
- 1 sweet potato, peeled and shredded
- 3 green onions, diced
- 10 eggs
- Freshly ground black pepper, to taste

Preparation

1. In an ovenproof skillet heat some oil over medium heat.
2. Add the sausages and cook till they get browned on all sides.
3. Now, add the sweet potatoes and cook till they become tender.
4. Add the green onions and sauté for about 2 minutes.

5. Pour the mixture into the greased skillet and swirls the skillet around to spread the batter in an even layer in the bottom of the pan.

6. Take a mixing bowl and whisk eggs in it. Pour this over the mixture in the pan.

7. Sprinkle pepper and let it cook for a bit or till the edges of the frittata are done.

8. Take the skillet off the stove and pop into an oven, preheated to 350 degrees F and bake until the frittata is cooked through.

9. Serve hot!

Delicious Italian Meatballs

Serves: 5

Ingredients

- 1/2 lb beef, ground
- 4 eggs, whisked
- 1 tsp dried oregano
- 1 lb pork, ground
- 4 garlic cloves, minced
- 1 lb veal, ground
- 4 tsp dried basil and parsley
- 1/2 cup almond flour
- 2 tsp salt and pepper
- 6 cups Italian sauce

Preparation

1. Keep the oven on preheat mode at 350 degrees F.

2. In a bowl combine together the ground beef, eggs, oregano, ground pork, cloves, ground veal, basil, parsley, almond flour, salt and pepper.

3. Knead the mixture with your hands until well combined and make 2-inch balls.

4. Grease a baking tray with some oil.

5. Place the prepared balls on a greased baking tray and bake them for around 20 or more minutes.

6. While the meatballs bake, pour the Italian sauce into a large pot and heat over a medium high flame till the sauce starts bubbling.

7. When done put them in the boiling pot of the sauce and cook for at least an hour.

8. Serve hot!

Zucchini Patties

Serves: 12

Ingredients

- 8 eggs, beaten
- 4 red bell peppers, roasted and finely diced
- 8 cups zucchini, grated
- 12 cloves of garlic, crushed
- 1 cup onion, chopped
- 2 tsp red pepper flakes
- 2 cup almond flour
- 3 tsp salt
- 8 tbsp olive oil

Preparation

1. Heat some oil in a skillet.

2. In a bowl add the eggs, bell pepper, zucchini, garlic, onion, red pepper flakes, almond flour and salt and whisk well to combine.

3. Pour one tablespoon of the mixture into the heated skillet and spread it around the bottom of the skillet. Try not to over spread it or your patties will have holes in them!

4. Cook for 3 minutes or so, flip and cook for another 3 minutes, or until evenly browned.

5. Repeat with the remaining batter and serve hot!

Chapter 10
Hashimoto's Disease and Workout

Living in this busy world, it is necessary to have time to yourself. At the end of a hectic day, you can be very tired. But it is very important for an individual to exercise to maintain a healthy lifestyle. Exercise will also help you increase your muscle strength and reduce the fatigue that you experience due to this disorder. Do not choose a very aggressive workout plan as it will leave you exhausted.

Also, people suffering from Hashimoto's thyroiditis often complain of an increase in weight, even when their appetite is poor. So it is essential to follow a workout program to avoid putting on unneeded pounds. Working out regularly will help you in losing excess weight. Unfortunately people suffering from the Hashimoto's disorder cannot regularly exercise because one of the most common and prevalent symptoms of the disorder is muscle pain and fatigue. To counter this you should talk to a professional gym instructor who can help you devise a good plan in accordance with your health. You should also contact your GP so that you do not start any new regime that might actually harm you.

Weak digestion is also noticed in individuals who suffer from this disease, exercising regularly helps in activating the metabolic activity of the body, thus further improving digestion. For digestion problems that are persistent you should contact a doctor as soon as possible.

Walking is the best-known exercise to lose weight. Start walking on a daily basis, initially walk for 30 minutes and then gradually increase your walking time to 1 hour per day. Make sure you walk at your own comfortable speed; after all, it is not a race. If you cannot walk continuously for 30 minutes, you can break the walk workout in 3 parts and walk for 10 minutes continuously thrice in a day. This will also help if you are on a strict schedule and do not get time to exercise regularly.

It may seem like a difficult thing to incorporate 3 10 minute walks in your daily schedule, but it is quite easy if you pay attention. Instead of taking a cab over short distances, you can walk or you can ask the cab to drop you a block away from your home and walk the rest of the distance.

Hashimoto's thyroiditis and yoga

Yoga is well known and popular form of exercise these days. Yoga acts on the body and the mind, helps calm your nerves, and aids in balancing out all the functions of the body. It also helps to refresh and calm your mind and thus frees you from stress - both physical and mental. Yoga helps in detoxifying the body.

"Yoga is the practice of quieting the mind." -Patanjali

The twisting and turning activity, which is done during yoga, indirectly helps in regulating blood all throughout the body. It helps in providing blood to each and every organ of the body so that they can function properly.

Yoga also helps in correcting and balancing the metabolism of the body, and thus can help you lose weight. One can control the symptoms of Hashimoto's Thyroiditis if they perform yoga on regular basis. Yoga helps you to heal your body internally and externally.

Meditation and the *pranayama* (breathing exercises) are also very helpful in controlling the disease and slowly aiding in curing it.

> Meditation will also help you to relax and forget about your ailments. It will also increase your concentration power and will help you calm down. Meditation also aids you in sleeping well and having dreamless sleep.

Hashimotos

Chapter 11
Dealing with Hashimoto's Thyroiditis as a Vegan

It can be difficult to deal with Hashimoto's as a vegan as you don't consume any animal products or animal byproducts. This chapter will throw light on how you can deal with Hashimoto's thyroiditis as a vegan.

As soon as you wake up, take the medicine that you are supposed to (mostly be vitamin supplements) and after that, take a glass of lemon water. Simply squeeze the juice of half a lemon into a glass of warm water. You can also add honey to this if you like. It is ideal to do this every day as it will get rid of the digestive discomfort that accompanies Hashimoto's Thyroiditis. It will also stimulate bowel movements and reduce the harmful effect of all the medicines you take. It also fights free radicals, clears your stomach from any impurities and neutralizes the stomach and fights fatigue. With this water you can add turmeric as it can help to reduce any inflammation. Turmeric is also an antibacterial and antiseptic and will let any lumps that are formed be healed naturally. Other spices that can be added include cinnamon, pepper or Siberian Ginseng. These are good for the thyroid gland and will improve your overall health and immunity.

Avoid consuming gluten foods as the protein component of it can bind to the thyroid glands, not letting it produce thyroid hormones. You can also go a step further and reduce the sugars in your food. Sugar can make you gain weight, which is common in people with thyroid disorders. Instead opt for sweeteners like coconut sugars, maple syrup and honey, as these are healthier. Also avoid consuming substances like hydrogenated oils, processed foods and so on. Whatever you take, take in moderation. Have chips once in a while, have alcohol once in a while but don't have them regularly. Plant based diets are extremely rich in fiber as opposed to meat based foods. They are also extremely healthy and nutritious and full of good cholesterol. If you are a meat eater, take baby steps to switch to vegetarian food and from then on vegan food. For instance, take smaller servings of meat and add more vegetables to your plate, opt for veggie burgers instead of meat patty ones and so on.

As far as goitrogenic food is concerned, it is important to consume them in small quantities. These vegetables and fruits can hamper the thyroid gland's iodine absorption and can also result in goiter. Foods like strawberries, kale, broccoli, peaches, soy, Brussels sprouts, cabbage, and millets and so on are very goitrogenic foods. They don't immediately cause goiter if you have a regular thyroid but they can result in your thyroid swelling up due to build up of tissue. Soy is something that should not be taken if you are susceptible to any kind of autoimmune disease. Eat it in limited quantities and don't eliminate it completely.

When it comes to breakfast, it's a good idea to have a green smoothie or a protein shake. Add some spinach leaves along with some ginger. You can also add beetroot which will give you relief and energy throughout the day. You can also take some hormone balancers after talking to your doctor about it. Take grains, cereals to incorporate carbohydrates. Take proteins in the form of lentils or beans and take some fat like nuts or seeds. While snacking, you can take some nuts and seeds and servings of good fruits. Try to avoid caffeine in the morning as it increases blood pressure. Coffee is not something that people with thyroid disorders should take because coffee acts much like how gluten acts in our body. It sticks to the thyroid glands and does not let the thyroid gland to secret the thyroid hormones. Apart from that, it reduces the efficiency of the thyroid gland and does not let it convert the inactive hormone T4 into active hormone T3. Caffeine can also cause the leaky gut syndrome and acid reflux. With Hashimoto's thyroiditis, the thyroid gland is highly inflamed and swollen and coffee aggravates this condition.

Get a metal detoxification if you can afford it. Metal poisoning can cause heavy problems with Hashimoto's Thyroiditis and can also lead to many other problems. Try going for liver cleansing and take foods like beetroot which help clean out the liver. Take lots of vitamin C rich foods like lemons and oranges and vitamin C supplements. Take a sauna every month and opt for doing yoga. Yoga is excellent for the thyroid, especially the pranayama. It reduces inflammation and stops excessive swelling. Go for a walk or look up other ways through which you can detoxify your body.

Remove all the amalgam fillers that are there in your teeth, with the help of a dentist, as they are the primary cause of metal poisoning. Do cardio workouts and go for a jog for fifteen minutes at least a day. Bask in the sun for ten minutes without using a sunscreen or a sun block. This will give your body adequate vitamin D. Vitamin D deficiency can also cause Hashimoto's Thyroiditis. It can also lead to brittle bones and much more. Try to get adequate sleep as well. Reduce late night parties and other activities, and give your body the rest it needs. Get 7 to 8 hours of sleep everyday as this will help nourish and heal the body. Make sure you have a nutrient rich diet and research how to have one efficiently. You can also consult your local nutritionist or dietitian for this purpose.

It is a common misconception that Hashimoto's Thyroiditis is not curable and you can't ever get rid of it but that is not true. With a few lifestyle changes and dietary changes you can get healthy thyroid glands. Perseverance is the key to long lasting happiness.

Chapter 12
Home Remedies for Hashimoto's Thyroiditis

In this chapter we look at some home remedies that will soothe and heal your condition.

Primrose Oil

The oil from primroses, especially the evening primrose variety, is helpful for combating thyroid related problems. It is very rich in GLA, also known as gamma linoleic acids, and thus helps in eradicating the inflammation that comes with Hashimoto's Thyroiditis. They also help in the production of thyroid hormones by stimulating the thyroid gland into functioning efficiently. They reduce the amount of hair loss that is associated with thyroid problems and can reduce heavy bleeding during menstruation. Simply add these in your salads and soups. You can also add a little in your milk.

Turmeric

Turmeric has been used since ancient times to reduce the effects of Hashimoto's Thyroiditis. This particular spice is commonly used in India and is used to reduce the inflammation that is associated with thyroid problems. It has a lot of medicinal properties and it also helps in detoxifying the body from harmful substances. It also aids in the functioning of the liver which is important for people with thyroid problems. It's even thought to reduce the size and danger of tumors. Try to add turmeric in your diet. You can add a teaspoon of turmeric in milk and drink this before going to bed. You can also make turmeric tea by adding a teaspoon of turmeric to hot water and add some lemon and honey and drink this.

Apple Cider Vinegar

Apple cider vinegar has several uses and it has a wide variety of benefits associated with it. It helps in detoxifying the body and in restoring the balance of acid and alkaline. It also helps you lose weight and regulates the hormones. It can increase your metabolism and increase immunity. Apple cider vinegar can also reduce the inflammation that is caused by Hashimoto's Thyroiditis. Add two tablespoons of apple cider vinegar to water and drink this every morning. You can also add a little bit of honey if you don't like the taste. Be sure to use organic apple cider vinegar as the regular ones may have a lot of harmful preservatives.

Ginger

Ginger is an all in all healing food that is an excellent source of zinc, potassium and manganese. These help in increasing immunity thereby reducing the severity of the condition. It also is excellent for thyroid related problems and can reduce inflammation. You can eat a small chunk of fresh ginger everyday. You can also add ginger into your usual dishes. Make ginger tea and drink it everyday. Simply boil water and add ginger to it. Add honey and lemon and drink this concoction everyday.

Fish Oils

The benefits of fish oils cannot be stressed enough. Fish oils contain huge amounts of DHA and EPA in their omega 3 fatty acids, which help in combating thyroid problems. They increase the metabolism of the thyroid gland and promote its healthy functioning. They also help to increase immunity and help combat inflammation caused by Hashimoto's Thyroiditis. Out of these, cod liver oil works the best and you can take a tablespoon of it every day. You can also get supplements of fish oil. However it is better to avoid taking these if you are on blood thinners and definitely consult your doctor before taking them.

Vitamin D

Vitamin D has been linked to thyroid problems and the most commonly associated with Hashimoto's Thyroiditis. Vitamin D deficiency could result in major problems like brittle bones, lowered immunity and so on. It is best to go out in the sun for about fifteen minutes everyday without sun block. Opt to go around the early morning time as the sun is a lot milder and there are less harmful UV rays present at this time. You can also do a few exercises in the sun that will stimulate the thyroid gland. Vitamin D will also reduce the inflammation and pains that are associated with Hashimoto's Thyroiditis.

Coconut Oil

Coconut is an excellent antifungal, antiseptic and antibacterial oil. This natural oil is excellent for soothing inflamed thyroid glands. It also helps to increase your metabolism and boosts your immune system to perform better thereby helping the thyroid glands to function properly. Those having Hashimoto's Thyroiditis usually have low basal body temperature. This particular oil helps in raising the temperature of the body, increasing the thyroid functions. Add two spoons of coconut oil to your milk and drink it in the morning. You can also add this to your smoothies. Also, simply substitute your regular oil for cooking for coconut oil. Be sure to use organically produced coconut oil or pure coconut oil.

Siberian Ginseng

Siberian Ginseng is a small woody shrub that is great for combating thyroid related problems. The leaves of this shrub can be used as herbs and can help with the production of the thyroid hormone. It also helps the thymus and adrenal gland perform better. It reduces fatigue and cures pains that come with Hashimoto's Thyroiditis. You can take a supplement of this by consulting your doctor or specialist.

Alternatively you can also add this herb to your salads, soups and dishes.

Guggul

Guggul is a type of resin from a variety of gum tree called Commiphora Mukul. This particular tree is most commonly found in India. It contains a particular substance called guggulsterones and studies have shown that these substances help to stimulate the thyroid gland and help it function smoothly. It has anti inflammation properties and hence reduces the inflammation that comes with Hashimoto's Thyroiditis. It is also used for several other thyroid related problems. You get these herbs in Indian shops and you can mix it with your salads and dishes. You can also take a supplement.

Vitamin B

Vitamin B has a variety of types and it is important to include as many varieties in your diet as possible. They are indispensable vitamins that will help in restoring the normalcy of the thyroid gland. Deficiency of vitamin B can cause Hashimoto's Thyroiditis. Take cereals, grains and vegetables and fruits to incorporate lots of vitamin B in your diet. You can also take a supplement. Simply ask your doctor and physician to recommend an appropriate supplement if necessary.

Chlorophyll

Chlorophyll is extremely important for those having Hashimoto's Thyroiditis and it helps in keeping the body safe from a malfunctioning thyroid gland. Chlorophyll contains lots of copper and this copper is important in oxygenating the body. When lots of oxygen is produced within the body, cell regeneration and cell growth improves. This will increase immunity and help in combating thyroid problems. It is best to supplement chlorophyll by drinking the juices of lots of green, leafy vegetables. Alternatively, add these leaves into salads, soups and dishes. You can also use chlorophyll by taking certain supplements.

Oysters

Raw oysters are one of the foods that is most rich in zinc. Zinc is very important for the immune system and is essential for those suffering from any form of thyroid problems including Hashimoto's Thyroiditis. This is because zinc can transform the compound or substance T4 into T3.

T3 is an active hormone while T4 is an inactive hormone. This transformation is not possible without the presence of zinc. Oysters also contain vitamin D which will help in reducing inflammation and pains associated with Hashimoto's Thyroiditis. In fact, deficiency of vitamin D is the most common cause of this disease. Have raw oyster or make oyster pancakes regularly.

Pears

Pears are super fruits that help to balance the hormones and hence are most commonly used in Chinese culture and recommended to those going through menopause or pregnancy. Pears are rich in fiber and thus they help flush out any antibodies or impurities that your body produces. They also help to neutralize any harmful reactions that take place within the body. They have huge amounts of vitamin E, C and B and also contain copper, which is required for the smooth functioning of the thyroid gland. It is a good idea to drink pear juice every day or have a small serving of pears every day.

Apples

Apples are similar to pears. They are extremely rich in essential nutrients and contain lots of fiber. The old saying "An apple day keeps the doctor away" is true. They help in detoxifying the body and getting rid of harmful byproducts. They also fight free radicals. They reduce amount of cholesterol you take in as a result of your diet. They also reduce constipation, which is a symptom of Hashimoto's Thyroiditis. They help in proper bowel movements and are rich in Vitamin A. They keep your mind active, preventing brain fog, and aid in preventing memory loss. Drink a glass of apple juice every day and have a few servings of apple each day. Apple and pear juice together would make a nutritious snack that would kill two birds with one stone.

Beetroot

Beetroot is excellent for the liver and is considered to be a liver detoxifier. A healthy liver is extremely important if you want your thyroid hormones to work efficiently. Studies have also shown that beetroot also contains phytonutrients, which are important for reducing the swelling of the thyroid gland and inflammation. It also reduces goiter and enlarged thyroid. The roots of the beets are more important as most nutrients are located there. They help in the smooth functioning of the bile duct. They also have anti inflammation and antioxidant properties and neutralize the harmful byproducts that are produced by the body.

Chapter 13
Myths Associated with Hashimoto's Thyroiditis

In this chapter, we will look at some of the myths that are associated with Hashimoto's Thyroiditis. Listed below are some of the most common myths and the truth relating to these questions.

Myth: Everyone who has the condition Hashimoto's Thyroiditis must be on thyroid hormones permanently.

Truth: Those who do have Hashimoto's Thyroiditis do not need to take thyroid hormones on permanent basis. This, again, depends upon the kind of condition that their thyroid gland is in. Those who need to take thyroid hormones permanently are those who have undergone thyroidectomy or those who have undergone radioactive iodine treatment. Those who haven't undergone any such treatment but have Hashimoto's Thyroiditis will have to take as many hormones as they need for as long as they need depending on the seriousness of their condition. However, this is impossible to know and so most doctors and specialists usually prescribe thyroid hormones permanently.

Myth: Those with Hashimoto's Thyroiditis will have to stop having all the gluten foods permanently.

Truth: This is also untrue. Avoiding gluten foods and eradicating gluten foods are two different things. While it is best to avoid gluten foods if you have the disorder, this is more important for those who have the leaky gut syndrome that is usually associated with it. Moderation is key and it is always better to switch to foods that are gluten free and there are a wide variety of these kinds of foods in the market. Usually the diet with respect to gluten foods depends upon the person; if the person is not sensitive then they can take gluten foods. But again, it must be noted that even for those who are not sensitive they may become sensitive over time.

Myth: Hashimoto's Thyroiditis is an autoimmune disease and hence there is no way one can be cured of it.

Truth: Though it is difficult to cure the condition, it is not impossible and there have been several success stories regarding this. Another aspect is scientists and researchers are constantly trying to work out ways through which they can cure these conditions. Natural treatments also work. Since Hashimoto's Thyroiditis is an autoimmune condition, there are several factors that can result in this condition. The key is to know which factor has been affecting the person. Stress, environmental factors, foods, genetics etc. all plays a very vital role in its development. If the factor has been identified, then treatment is a lot easier. Though people cannot fix a genetic factor, environment and lifestyle choices can be changed and therefore treat the disorder.

Myth: People with Hashimoto's Thyroiditis should not take iodine.

Truth: The topic of iodine is widely discussed and debated since the discovery of Hashimoto's Thyroiditis. This is because iodine creates an oxidative reaction with the thyroid hormones which can damage the thyroid glands and trigger an autoimmune response. Those who do happen to take iodine should also take selenium along with magnesium and vitamin C as well. Selenium and vitamin C will help to eradicate the oxidation process while magnesium helps in absorbing the excess iodine that is present. However, it is important to note that everyone requires some form of iodine in the body for functioning of several organs and glands.

Myth: Cruciferous vegetables should be eradicated from the diets of people with Hashimoto's Thyroiditis.

Truth: This is also not true. However, it should be noted that these vegetables should not be consumed in excess. They also supply essential vitamins and minerals that are required by the body to work. Avoiding these does not cause any harm and tiny doses of these help to stimulate the thyroid gland into functioning. You can have a small servings of these every day and not hinder your health. There have been several studies conducted on this topic and currently extensive research is being done on these vegetables and fruits to link them to Hashimoto's Thyroiditis.

Myth: The TSH Test is the Best Test for Thyroid Disease

Truth: Most people have been diagnosed with this disorder after only being tested with the TSH test. It is important to note that this test is not a comprehensive test. Though it is a requirement and shows many details, this test is based on the blood profile of the person and may not be able to detect any thyroid abnormality. It is best to get a few more tests done to know the condition of your thyroid gland, especially if you are facing severe symptoms and your TSH test came negative for thyroid. Some tests include the Free T4, Reverse T3, Thyroid Peroxidase Antibodies, Free T3, and Thyroid Stimulating Immunoglobulins and so on. These tests are the ones that usually throw light on hypothyroidism, hyperthyroidism and Hashimoto's Thyroiditis.

Myth: All thyroid lumps or nodules are automatically cancerous

Truth: Not even 10 per cent of all the thyroid lumps or nodules are cancerous. It is important to note that the lumps that are formed in the thyroid glands are usually not cancerous but exposure to radiation especially from microwaves and other such environmental factors can turn the lumps into cancerous ones. Usually, the lumps or nodules are not dealt with if they don't cause you any discomfort. If they do, then there is always the possibility of treatment or surgery that is done to remove these lumps.

Myth: All the natural thyroid supplements that are prescribed usually don't work.

Truth: In fact, this is the opposite. Regular medicines that are given to treat thyroid like Levothyroxine and so on do not contain all the essential compounds and substances that the thyroid gland requires. They only contain T4, which is only one of the many small substances that your thyroid gland requires for smooth functioning. Natural supplements like Nature Thyroid, Erfa and so on contain both T3 and T4, which are essential to stimulate the thyroid gland.

Myth: Men usually do not acquire Hashimoto's Thyroiditis or any other thyroid problems.

Truth: Men are at a lower risk of developing thyroid problems however there are several cases where men do acquire them. In fact, statistics show that 2 in 10 men acquire some form of thyroid problems in their lives. The symptoms and severity of the thyroid problems however are usually much less than women. Those with higher levels of estrogen are more at risk for thyroid problems.

Myth: It is not possible to lose weight due to Hashimoto's Thyroiditis

Truth: It is definitely more difficult to lose weight due to Hashimoto's Thyroiditis but it not impossible. This is because the disorder results in sluggish thyroid glands and this in turn reduces your body's efficiency to burn calories. It is common to think you are gaining weight but you need to realize that you are usually not gaining weight but it appears so because you are losing weight at a much slower rate than normal. But with adequate exercises, a low carbohydrate diet and healthier options, it is certainly possible to lose weight quickly.

Veronica Baruwal

Chapter 14
Tips and Points to be Noted

There are always some dos and don't when you are suffering from Hashimoto's Thyroiditis. This chapter throws light on some of the tips and points that you should note when you are suffering from Hashimoto's Thyroiditis. Listed below are a few of those points to remember.

1. Do not use non-stick cookware. It is best to get rid of all your non-stick cookware. Research and several studies have shown that non-stick cookware contains a particular substance called perfluorooctanoic acid, or PFOA, which is linked to thyroid problems. In fact, it is said to double the risk of getting thyroid related problems. The studies show that those with Hashimoto's Thyroiditis have a higher

concentration of this compound in their blood. It can lead to poor effectiveness of the gland.

2. Eliminate soy. Soy contains compounds that will reduce the natural functions that the thyroid gland does. Thus it results in an imbalance of hormones and can complicate Hashimoto's Thyroiditis by enlarging the thyroid gland bringing about goiter. It also disrupts the usage of iodine Another issue with soy is that it will hinder the absorption of thyroid supplements that are prescribed to you.

3. Remember to follow an alkaline diet. Alkaline diets are not just important for people who suffer from Hashimoto's Thyroiditis but for everyone. This is because this particular form of diet will prevent bone demineralization, muscle pain, back pain, kidney stones, asthma etc. Following an alkaline diet will reduce excessive thyroid activity. Alkaline diets do not mean cutting down on all acidic food because acidic food gives you the nutrients that you require. It is best to increase alkaline foods such as certain fruits and vegetables in your diet in proportion to the amount of acidic food that you consume.

4. Do not forget to exercise. Now, it is best to consult a physician or a specialist to find out what kind of exercise is right for you because certain exercises may be harmful with your condition. However, that does not mean you do not exercise. Exercising will result in the production of more growth hormones. It will increase your immunity and will increase the insulin reception of your body. This in fact is one of the primary causes of Hashimoto's Thyroiditis. It is also a good idea to exercise 10 minutes after you wake up as this will increase the benefits.

5. If you are suffering from Hashimoto's Thyroiditis, be sure to take steps and necessary action to balance your estrogen levels. This is because excessive estrogen in the body will slow down the functioning of the thyroid gland. If you are on birth control pills and medications, it is best to visit a gynecologist so they can assess the impact they may have on your health. Opt to eat vegetarian or plant based diets as they have higher fiber content in them. It is also advisable to reduce the amount of dairy you consume because dairy consists of high amounts of estrogen. It is best to avoid non-organic meats as well because of the high content of growth hormones present in these meats.

6. Eat foods that are rich in tyrosine. Tyrosine is one of the amino acids that is produced by foods such as fish, yogurt, cheese, turkey, bananas, avocados, peanuts, almonds, pumpkin seeds and so on. These amino acids help the cells of the body to synthesize proteins. Thus, this natural amino acid helps people to produce their own thyroid hormone. Another benefit of this is that it combats the depression that may accompany Hashimoto's Thyroiditis. Ask your physician or a specialist for recommendations regarding the dosage. A famous tablet that is commonly used is the L-Tyrosine, which can be taken twice a day.

7. Take foods that are rich in arginine. Arginine is another amino acid. It is one of the 20 amino acids that are found naturally. These amino acids are present in foods such as milk, yogurt, cheese, seafood like fishes, lobsters, shrimp, chicken, quails, peanuts, pumpkin seeds and so on. These help in cell division and increase the production of hormones, one of them being the thyroid hormone. Another important benefit of this amino acid is that it helps in removing ammonia in the body. Thus, it helps in the smooth functioning of the thyroid gland. A popular form of arginine

comes in the form of L-arginine, which can be taken for those suffering from Hashimoto's Thyroiditis.

8. Avoid consuming goods and foods that contain fluoride. Fluoride is one of the reasons for the onset of Hashimoto's Thyroiditis and this particular compound can reduce the efficiently of the thyroid gland. It also suppresses the functions of the thyroid gland by not letting it produce the thyroid hormone. It is best to avoid sources that contain this compound such as tea ad coffee wherein fluoride is naturally present. Try using fluoride free toothpaste and avoid drinking soft drinks and aerated beverages. Use a shower filter because the water that comes to our homes is treated and may have high levels of fluoride in it. Also avoid meat and opt for vegetarian or vegan diets.

9. Consume foods that have low mercury levels. This implies that it is necessary to consume low mercury seafood. This is because mercury is a very heavy metal and will stick to the thyroid gland, hampering its functions and hindering the production of thyroid hormones. Fish such as tuna, swordfish and some types of sharks are considered to be extremely high on mercury and it is best to completely avoid

them. If you have mercury fillings in your teeth it is best to go to your dentist and get them replaced. Mercury also does not allow the conversion of certain compounds, like that of T4 to T3, which can cause problems.

10. It is best to avoid excessive consumption of vegetable oils especially canola oil. This is simply because canola oil is an unsaturated fatty oil and this reduces the production of thyroid hormones by the thyroid gland. Unsaturated oils promote inflammation. They contain substances like omega-6 fatty acid, which can hamper the functions of the thyroid glands. It also contains MSG, which can affect the thyroid glands.

11. Bisphenol A is a chemical compound and a form of synthetic carbon. It is commonly referred to as BPA and is found in plastic bottles and plastic containers. This particular compound is known to block the thyroid hormone receptors. It is known to disrupt the thyroid and estrogen endocrine, thus affecting the thyroid glands in their regular functioning. It binds into the receptors and suppresses the functions of the glands. It is found that people with Hashimoto's Thyroiditis have high concentrations of BPA in

their systems. Thus it is always better to drink out of stainless steel bottles or paper cups. Avoid the plastic lids on top of coffee containers as well.

12. Remember to eat foods that are rich in omega 3s. These are fatty acids that are extremely beneficial, especially for those suffering from thyroid problems. It helps in reducing the inflammation of the thyroid glands. It also helps in faster recovery by boosting the immune system. Thereby, it also reduces the severity of the condition. The ratio of omega 3 fatty acids to omega 6 fatty acids should usually be equal to ensure smooth functioning of the thyroid gland. Omega 3 fatty acids are found in food like milk, cream, cheese, ducks, fish, organically grown eggs, chicken, and lamb. You can also ask your physician or specialist to prescribe you some omega 3 supplements.

13. It is a good idea to have some form of fish oil. This is because fish oils contain huge amounts of omega 3 fatty acids. But apart from just these, they have the highest content of substances like DHA and EPA in the fatty acids. DHA is used to support the brain during Hashimoto's Thyroiditis and will reduce the severity of the autoimmune

disease. These will reduce mood swings, depression, and brain fog and so on, which are caused by Hashimoto's Thyroiditis. EPA will reduce the pain aches and swelling that is accompanied by the disorder. If you are a vegetarian or a vegan and you cannot take a fish oil, take substances like avocados, olive oil, raw nuts and pumpkin seeds.

14. Goitrogenic vegetables are vegetables that high in goitrogens, which are substances, which interfere with the regular functioning of the thyroid gland. They release antibodies against the thyroid, which will hinder all processes, including the release of the enzymes thyroid peroxidase. These enzymes are required in order to bring iodine to the thyroid to help it function. Hence, it is imperative to cook or boil goitrogenic vegetables before consuming them. These processes will kill the excess amounts of goitrogens that are present in these vegetables, which will reduce the negative effects. Some examples of these vegetables include kale, cauliflower, turnips, sprouts and broccoli.

15. Additional to every other fish oil that you take, it is best to take a spoon of fermented cod liver oil everyday. Apart

from being one of the best sources of omega 3 fatty acids, it is also consists vitamin A and vitamin D which are important for detoxifying your body especially from mercury. They will reduce the pain and excess swelling caused by Hashimoto's Thyroiditis. They also will enable the smooth functioning of the thyroid glands because of the high concentration of eicosapentaenoic acid (EPA) and docosahexaenoic acid (DHA). They will also reduce arthritis, especially rheumatoid arthritis.

16. It is also a good idea to take a small brisk walk without sunscreen in the mornings. Get some sun. Sunlight helps reduce the inflammation that is associated with Hashimoto's Thyroiditis. It will also provide abundant amounts of vitamin D, which will get hindered by a sunscreen or a sun block. This will enable the smooth functioning of the thyroid gland. The benefit of going out in the sun is that the natural sunlight enables the body to produce Vitamin D. In fact, it is possible to produce about 10,000 IUs of vitamin D in one day by our body. This vitamin is very important as it helps to control your immune system and increase its efficiency. It also reduces the risk of acquiring several conditions and helps reducing the time to taken to cure autoimmune

diseases like Hashimoto's Thyroiditis. Try to spend at least 15 minutes out in the sun each day.

17. Try to remove the excessive amount of processed foods from your diet. This is because processed foods contain huge amounts of goitrogens, which can affect the production of the thyroid hormone by the thyroid gland. They also contain huge amounts of sugars, trans fats and hydrogenated oils. It is best to consume organically produced foods, which do not contain pesticides and other harmful chemicals, as otherwise you can slow the functions of the thyroid glands and increase the inflammation. This will allow your body to heal and become nourished with good vitamins and minerals. Take plenty of fruits and vegetables; opt for purified water over aerated beverages, herbal teas and unsweetened yogurt, flax seed and so on. It is also important to cut down on refined goods, such as refined sugar and so on.

18. Start dry brushing at least once in two days. Dry brushing is a very effective technique and is called Garshana in Ayurveda. It was first started in India several centuries ago. This particular technique is very effective as it helps to

stimulate the lymphatic system and helps in draining the excessive amounts of lymph that is produced by the body. It also helps in the body's natural healing process by getting rid of toxins. Apart from all these, it also promotes blood circulation and promotes the regeneration of the cells. Alternately you can also alternate between dry brushing and cold rinses. You can look up various ways to do this and it is most beneficial if done in the morning after you wake up.

19. It is a good idea to incorporate grass fed gelatin into your diet. Gelatin is considered to be a super food especially for those suffering from Hashimoto's Thyroiditis. It is extremely good for the digestive tract, heart, liver, skin and muscles. It is believed to also increased the efficiency of the immune system. Apart from just these, it helps in detoxifying the body. When you are purchasing gelatin, ensure you buy organic gelatin and also ensure that the gelatin does not contain MSG.

20. Ensure that you take adequate amounts of saturated fats. Saturated fats are those, which have several functions. However be sure not to take more than 20 grams of it every day. Organic saturated fats are found in substances like lard,

coconut oil and so on. They help to reduce the inflammation of the thyroid glands and in crease the metabolism of the body. Another great benefit of saturated fats is that they improve brain activity and combat brain related problems caused by Hashimoto's Thyroiditis like memory loss, brain fog and so on. They also help in proper nerve signaling. This will result in greater efficiency of the neurons and these neurons will help improve the functioning of the thyroid gland.

21. Fermented foods like sauerkraut; kimchi, cultured vegetables, condiments and fish have huge amounts of good bacteria. These good bacterial are excellent sources of fiber and are excellent for the digestive tract. With Hashimoto's Thyroiditis you can experience leaky gut. This condition is the intestinal permeability wherein you suffer from acid reflux, troubled bowels, stomach pains, cramps and so on. Hence taking probiotics will prevent this. Another great thing about probiotics is that it reduces the amount of ulcers that can be caused by autoimmune diseases like Hashimoto's Thyroiditis. Additionally you can take probiotics like yogurt and probiotic shakes as well or ask

your physician or specialist to suggest a probiotic supplement for your diet.

22. Reduce the amount of carbohydrates that you take per day. This is important because too many carbohydrates can increase the estrogen that the body produces and estrogen can affect the functioning of the thyroid gland. Consume foods like coconut milk, coconut oil, flaxseeds, hemp seeds, avocado, and salmon and so on.

23. Increase the amount of selenium in your diet. However, take them in moderate quantities. Consume foods like salmon, beef, mushrooms, sunflower seeds, onions and so on. Selenium reduces the amount of iodine produced by the thyroid gland. It will dilute the iodine which reduces the effects. It also promotes the well-being of the thyroid gland.

24. Reduce the amount of gluten and A1 casein. These substances can cause a condition that is a symptom of thyroid problems called leaky gut. Also the molecular structure that is found in the protein parts of these substances resembled the thyroid gland. When you consume gluten substances, the gliadin crosses the blood barrier entering the bloodstream and hence starts producing

antibodies to attack the thyroid gland. It will also interfere with your medication.

Conclusion

As you can see from this book Hashimoto's Thyroiditis is an autoimmune disorder where the immune cells attack the thyroid gland by causing severe inflammation in the area. This then results in the impairment of the thyroid gland and production of insufficient quantities of the thyroid hormone.

Do not panic if you are diagnosed with Hashimoto's Thyroiditis. This disease is absolutely treatable. Individuals who suffer from this disease need to understand that they should be aware of all the symptoms of the disease so that they are in control of the situation and do not panic at the onset of a new symptom. If you are suffering from Hashimoto's Thyroiditis and suddenly experience a slowdown in speech, you may panic, thinking that something is majorly wrong, when this is just another symptom of your prevalent disease. In order to avoid this sort of panic, it is essential that you study your disease well.

Thank you once again for choosing this book, and I hope you find it beneficial to combating this disease.

Disclaimer: Do not consume any medicine or drug without consulting with your physician. This applies to all the drugs mentioned in this book.

www.ingramcontent.com/pod-product-compliance
Lightning Source LLC
Chambersburg PA
CBHW051907170526
45168CB00001B/275